Emergencies in Diabetes

Emergencies in Diabetes

Diagnosis, Management and Prevention

Editor

Andrew J. Krentz

Southampton University Hospitals, UK

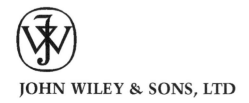

JOHN WILEY & SONS, LTD

Other Wiley Editorial Offices

John Wiley & Sons, Inc., 111 River Street, Hoboken, NJ 07030, USA

Jossey-Bass, 989 Market Street, San Francisco, CA 94103-1741, USA

Wiley-VCH Verlag GmbH, Boschstrasse 12, D-69469 Weinheim, Germany

John Wiley & Sons Australia Ltd, 33 Park Road, Milton, Queensland 4064, Australia

John Wiley & Sons (Asia) Pte Ltd, 2 Clementi Loop #02-01, Jin Xing Distripark, Singapore 129809

John Wiley & Sons (Canada) Ltd, 22 Worcester Road, EtobicokeRexdale, Ontario, Canada M9W 1L1

Wiley also publishes its books in a variety of electronic formats. Some content that appears in print
may not be available in electronic books.

Library of Congress Cataloging-in-Publication Data

   Emergencies in diabetes : diagnosis, management and prevention / editor, Andrew J. Krentz.
      p.   cm.
   Includes bibliographical references and index.
   ISBN 0-471-49814-9 (pbk. : alk. paper)
   1. Diabetes–Complications.   2. Medical emergencies.
      [DNLM: 1. Diabetes Mellitus–complications.   2. Emergencies. WK 835 E53 2004]
   I. Krentz, Andrew J.
   RC660 .E44   2004
   616.4'62025–dc22   2004000702

British Library Cataloguing in Publication Data
A catalogue record for this book is available from the British Library

ISBN 0-471-49814-9

Typeset in 10.5/13 pt. Palatino by Thomson Press (India) Ltd, New Delhi
Printed and bound in Great Britain by TJ International Ltd., Padstow, Cornwall
This book is printed on acid-free paper responsibly manufactured from sustainable forestry
in which at least two trees are planted for each one used for paper production.

Contents

Preface

Diabetes mellitus can usually be reasonably well controlled on a day-to-day basis with modern drug regimens. Nonetheless, the risks of metabolic decompensation and iatrogenic hypoglycaemia remain close at hand. Life threatening hyperglycaemia – with or without ketosis – may be precipitated by intercurrent illness or interruption of antidiabetic therapy; new cases of diabetes frequently present as hyperglycaemic emergencies. Clinical outcomes for patients with diabetes after myocardial infarction or surgery may be compromised by sub-optimal metabolic control, the presence of chronic co-morbidity in the form of microvascular complications or atherosclerosis magnifying these risks. Pregnancy continues to present particular hazards for mother and fetus.

Considerable evidence has now accumulated pointing to the prospect of improved outcomes for more patients with diabetes through meticulous attention to clinical care. Inevitably, many patients will experience temporary periods of metabolic instability that can be difficult to manage even in a controlled hospital environment. Experienced clinicians will attest to the challenges often presented by patients with diabetic metabolic emergencies.

This book has been written by experienced authors and investigators, each an expert in his or her field. The chapters aspire to present the salient features of each emergency in an accessible format. We hope the book will be of value to a range of health care professionals who care for patients with diabetes.

AJK
Southampton, UK
February 2004

Contributors

Aftab M. Ahmad, MD
Department of Medicine
Royal Liverpool Hospital
Prescott Street
Liverpool L7 8XP
UK

Mark R. Burge, MD
University of New Mexico
    School of Medicine
Department of Medicine/
    Endocrinology – 5ACC
Albuquerque, NM 87131
USA

Kathleen M. Colleran, MD
University of New Mexico
    School of Medicine
Department of Medicine/
    Endocrinology – 5ACC
Albuquerque, NM 87131
USA

David B. Dunger, MD FRCP
Department of Paediatrics
Box 116, University of Cambridge
Addenbrooke's Hospital
Cambridge CB2 2QQ
UK

Julie A. Edge
Paediatric Department
The John Radcliffe
Headington, Oxford OX3 9DU
UK

John E. Gerich, MD
University of Rochester School
    of Medicine
Department of Medicine
Rochester, NY 14642
USA

Simon R. Heller, DM FRCP
Clinical Sciences Centre
Northern General Hospital
Sheffield S5 7AU
UK

**Helen B. Holt,
MB ChB MRCP (UK)**
Southampton University
    Hospitals NHS Trust
Southampton SO16 6YD
UK

Andrew J. Krentz,
MD FRCP
Southampton University
   Hospitals NHS Trust
Southampton SO16 6YD
UK

Jean-Daniel Lalau, MD
Service d'Endocrinologie-
   Nutrition
Hôpital Sud
Amiens
France

Jiten P. Vora
Department of Medicine
Royal Liverpool Hospital
Prescott Street
Liverpool L7 8XP
UK

Hans J. Woerle, MD
Ludwig-Maximilians-
   University of Munich
Department of Internal
   Medicine II
Munich
Germany

1

Diabetic Ketoacidosis in Adults

Andrew J Krentz and **Helen B Holt**

Summary

Diabetic ketoacidosis has a reported average mortality of approximately five per cent in Western countries. Mortality is generally higher at the extremes of age.

Common precipitating causes include infection, insulin management errors, omission of insulin and new cases of diabetes; in many cases no cause is obvious.

Although traditionally considered uncommon in patients with type 2 diabetes, reports in recent years have drawn attention to diabetic ketoacidosis in non-white patients who are often able to discontinue insulin after recovery.

Ketoacidosis develops when there is an absolute or, more commonly, a relative insulin deficiency, usually in concert with an increase in catabolic hormone concentrations. Hepatic overproduction of glucose and ketone bodies is compounded by diminished clearance in peripheral tissues.

Emergencies in Diabetes   Edited by Andrew J. Krentz
© 2004 John Wiley & Sons, Ltd   ISBN 0-471-49814-9

Classical symptoms include increasing polyuria and polydipsia, acute weight loss, generalised weakness, drowsiness and, in approximately l0 per cent of cases, eventual coma; abdominal pain is recognised, particularly in younger patients. Physical signs including dehydration, hypotension, tachycardia, hyperventilation and hypothermia are usually prominent in more severe cases. Any patient in whom the diagnosis is suspected should be promptly admitted to hospital.

Initial investigations should include measurement of capillary blood glucose and urinary or plasma ketone estimation by reagent strips; these, in the context of the clinical features, should be sufficient to confirm the diagnosis. Bedside tests should be confirmed by laboratory measurements of blood glucose, urea, Na^+, K^+, Cl^- desirable but not essential, full blood count (arterial blood pH and gases in shocked patients) in conjunction with appropriate cultures of blood, urine etc.

Treatment comprises the following.

Rehydration. Initially with isotonic saline (e.g. 1 L/h for first 2–3 h, totalling 6–10 L for first 24 h); 5 per cent dextrose 1 L 4–6 hourly is substituted for saline when blood glucose has fallen to ≤15 mmol/L; dextrose (+ insulin) is continued until the patient is drinking and eating.

Short-acting insulin. This should be given by intravenous infusion, e.g. 5–10 U/h until blood glucose reaches ≤15 mmol/L; the infusion rate is subsequently reduced, typically to 1–4 U/h in order to maintain capillary blood glucose between 5 and 10 mmol/L. Insulin requirements at this point are affected by insulin resistance (exacerbated in ketoacidosis) and adequacy of rehydration. Subcutaneous insulin is (re)commenced when the patient starts eating again, intravenous insulin being discontinued at this point. Insulin therapy should not be interrupted during treatment of ketoacidosis.

Potassium replacement. If normokalaemia is present and renal function is normal, ~20 mmol potassium chloride is added to each litre of infusate; the dose of potassium chloride is adjusted by careful monitoring of serum potassium concentrations.

Sodium bicarbonate. Rarely indicated. Small doses, i.e. 100 mmol, given as 1.26 per cent solution, may be considered if arterial pH < 7.0 or if cardio-respiratory collapse appears imminent.

Complications. In adults, respiratory distress syndrome may be encountered, especially if rehydration has been over-zealous. Cerebral oedema is largely confined to paediatric practice. Thrombo-embolic complications require anti-coagulation. Rhino-cerebral mucormycosis is rare.

Introduction

Diabetic ketoacidosis continues to be an important cause of morbidity and mortality in patients with type 1 diabetes. All episodes are, at least theoretically, avoidable since administration of sufficient doses of insulin should avert major metabolic decompensation. However, many cases occur because of dosing errors or discontinuation of insulin therapy; some patients, perhaps understandably, seem to find it difficult to adjust their insulin regimens appropriately during illness.

> Diabetic ketoacidosis remains an important cause of death among patients with type 1 diabetes

Although it principally affects younger patients with type 1 diabetes, ketoacidosis may be precipitated in patients with type 2 diabetes during severe intercurrent illness. Recent reports from the USA and Asia have highlighted the difficulties in classifying non-white patients as having type 1 or type 2 diabetes by a history of ketoacidosis. Ketoacidosis is occasionally the presenting feature of type 1 diabetes in the elderly. In the USA, socio-economic factors and difficulties in access to care may lead to discontinuation of insulin among poor urban blacks. The annual total cost of hospitalisations in the USA because of diabetic ketoacidosis may exceed $100 million. Reports in the literature provide little evidence that hospitalisation rates for diabetic ketoacidosis have declined in recent decades.

Definition

The cardinal biochemical features of diabetic ketoacidosis are hyperketonaemia and metabolic acidosis, in concert with variable hyperglycaemia. While no univerally agreed criteria for diagnosis exist, diabetic ketoacidosis may be defined as in Box 1.1.

Box 1.1 Definition of diabetic ketoacidosis

- Severe uncontrolled diabetes requiring emergency treatment with insulin and intravenous fluids

- Blood total ketone body concentration, i.e. the sum of acetoacetate and 3-hydroxybutyrate $\geq$ 5 mmol/L.

Note that biochemical confirmation of the diagnosis is often based on semi-quantitative urine dipstick methods, a minority of centres having clinical chemistry laboratories that can measure blood ketone body concentrations. The diagnostic criteria that we use are presented in Box 1.2. Note that no threshold for hyperglycaemia is included in this definition, reflecting the wide variability in blood glucose concentrations.

Box 1.2 Practical biochemical definition of diabetic ketoacidosis

- Blood bicarbonate concentration (capillary or arterial) $\leq$ 15 mmol/L

- Significant ketosis, defined as urine Ketostix® (Bayer Diagnostics) reaction ++ or plasma Ketostix® + or more).

Mortality

Diabetic ketoacidosis continues to be an important cause of death among patients with type 1 diabetes. The average mortality rate for ketoacidosis today is quoted as between 5 and 10 per cent although rates vary widely. Experienced centres would expect to report a mortality rate of less than five per cent. Some deaths are inevitable consequences of associated medical conditions such as overwhelming infection. Clearly, the mortality associated with diabetic ketoacidosis has not been abolished, despite the ready availability of insulin, at least in Western countries. Mortality rates for diabetic ketoacidosis vary with prevailing socio-economic factors and the provision of general medical care.

- *Developing countries.* In Tanzania during the 1980s, for example, hospital mortality rates from ketoacidosis were reminiscent of those during the pre-insulin era in the West.

- *Industrialised countries.* Even in countries with well developed health care systems some deaths associated with ketoacidosis are potentially preventable, arising from factors such as

  o delays in presentation or diagnosis

  o errors in management, either by the patient on the part of medical attendants.

Differences in (1) the definition of ketoacidosis and (2) patient selection may also account for a proportion of this variation. Mortality need not be higher in non-university hospitals than in teaching centres if appropriate guidelines for management are implemented. Mortality is generally higher in certain groups of patients such as the very elderly.

Precipitating factors

- *Infection.* This is the commonest identifiable cause of ketoacidosis reported in the literature, accounting for approximately 35 per cent of all episodes, pneumonia and urinary tract infections being the most frequent types.

- *New cases of diabetes.* These account for approximately 10–15 per cent of episodes.

- *Management errors.* These include inappropriate changes in insulin dosage initiated either by the patient or sometimes following medical advice.

- *Recurrent ketoacidosis.* This affects a small subgroup of patients, the majority being females under the age of 20 years in whom psychological problems lead to discontinuation of insulin.

- *Other factors.* No precipitating cause is identified in approximately 25–35 per cent of episodes, although this depends on the rigour with which the search is conducted. Ultimately, it must be concluded that insufficient insulin has been administered.

Higher rates of ketoacidosis have been observed in some centres specialising in continuous subcutaneous insulin infusion (CSII). In the Diabetes Control and Complications Trial (DCCT), a higher rate of ketoacidosis was observed in patients receiving CSII than in those on multiple insulin injections. It has been suggested that the small subcutaneous depot of regular insulin in CSII predisposes to the rapid development of ketoacidosis if the infusion is interrupted.

> Discontinuation of insulin treatment is a common cause of diabetic ketoacidosis

Pathogenesis

Diabetic ketoacidosis is characterised by marked elevations of catabolic counter-regulatory hormone concentrations:

- glucagon

- catecholamines

- cortisol

- growth hormone.

These increases, often in concert with elevated levels of inflammatory cytokines, occur in the presence of an absolute or relative deficiency of insulin. While insulin may be measurable in plasma it is, by definition, insufficient to maintain a normal metabolic state. Insulin resistance, a reduced biological action of the hormone, is acutely increased in diabetic ketoacidosis, compounding any deficiency in circulating insulin. In patients with type 2 diabetes, residual endogenous insulin secretion serves to protect against ketoacidosis (see Chapter 3). However, suppression of β-cell insulin secretion by catecholamines (via α-adrenergic receptors) may occasionally precipitate ketoacidosis during acute severe illness; this may be especially true of patients with type 2 diabetes of long duration in whom β-cell function may be more compromised. A practical rule of thumb is to regard any patient with insulin-treated diabetes as having major insulin deficiency. This has implications for the management of diabetes during severe intercurrent illness, trauma and surgery (see Chapter 7).

> Severe intercurrent illness may precipitate ketoacidosis in patients with type 2 diabetes.

Under experimental conditions, withdrawal of insulin from insulin-dependent patients leads to an early rise in plasma glucagon. As hyperglycaemia and ketoacidosis develop, progressive dehydration and acidosis stimulate the release of catecholamines (adrenaline and nor-adrenaline) and cortisol. A vicious circle develops in which worsening metabolic decompensation stimulates further secretion of catabolic hormones. Hepatic overproduction of glucose and ketone bodies initiates hyperglycaemia and ketosis, while impaired disposal by peripheral tissues such as muscle and brain maintains and exacerbates hyperglycaemia and hyperketonaemia. The rate of glucose production subsequently decreases towards normal but hyperglycaemia is maintained as the rates of production and utilisation become equal. Insulin withdrawal also results in a progressive increase in ketone body production and utilization. However, the former exceeds the latter, resulting in a progressive rise in plasma ketone bodies.

Insulin deficiency with elevated counter-regulatory hormones initiates hyperglycaemia and ketosis

---

We will now consider the biochemical disturbances in more detail.

- *Hyperglycaemia.* Insulin deficiency and elevated plasma levels of catabolic hormones, particularly glucagon and catecholamines, result in increased rates of hepatic glycogenolysis and gluconeogenesis; in addition, renal gluconeogenesis is enhanced by acidosis, although it contributes quantitatively less to hyperglycaemia. Glucose disposal by tissues such as skeletal muscle and adipocytes is reduced by insulin deficiency; elevated plasma levels of catabolic hormones and non-esterified fatty acids with acidosis induce insulin resistance.

- *Hyperketonaemia.* In ketoacidosis, serum ketone body levels are often raised to 200–300 times their normal fasting values. Ketone bodies are strong organic acids that are fully dissociated at physiological pH. In turn, this results in equimolar generation of hydrogen ions (H^+) outstripping the buffering capacity of fluids and tissues. Metabolic acidosis has a number of serious detrimental physiological effects that account for many of the serious clinical features of ketoacidosis:

o negative inotropic effect on cardiac muscle

o exacerbation of systemic hypotension through peripheral vasodilatation

o exacerbation of insulin resistance

o increased risk of ventricular arrhythmias

o respiratory depression with severe acidosis.

Ketogenesis

Insulin deficiency and catabolic hormone excess, especially of catecholamines, promote lipolysis within adipocytes, wherein triglycerides are converted to three fatty acids and one molecule of glycerol. These effects are mediated via the activity of hormone-sensitive lipase (triacylglycerol lipase), an enzyme normally regarded as being exquisitely sensitive to inhibition by insulin. Concurrently, re-esterification, i.e. the formation of new triglycerides, within adipocytes is impaired. This results in the net release of long-chain non-esterified fatty acids and glycerol into the circulation (Figure 1.1).

Glycerol is a gluconeogenic precursor while fatty acids are the principal substrate for ketone bodies. Hepatic ketogenesis is enhanced by increased portal delivery of fatty acids liberated from adipocyte stores. In diabetic ketoacidosis, hepatic re-esterification of fatty acids is impaired and fatty acids are preferentially partially oxidised to ketone bodies within mitochondria (Figure 1.2).

1. Fatty acids are converted to coenzyme A (CoA) derivatives prior to transportation into mitochondria by an active transport system (the carnitine shuttle). The hormonal imbalance in diabetic ketoacidosis, i.e. insulin deficiency and excess catabolic hormones, favours entry of fatty acids into the mitochondria. This is mediated via a glucagon-mediated decrease in the

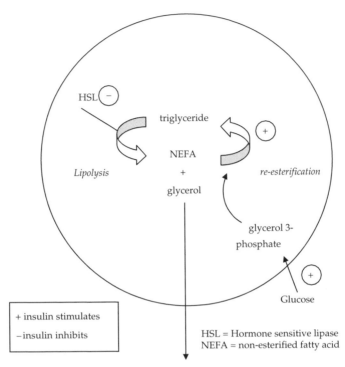

+ insulin stimulates

−insulin inhibits

HSL = Hormone sensitive lipase
NEFA = non-esterified fatty acid

Figure 1.1   Effects of insulin on mobilisation of fatty acids from adipocytes

cytosolic concentration of malonyl-CoA (via reduced conversion of pyruvate to acetyl coenzyme A), a potent competitive inhibitor of carnitine-palmitoyl transferase I. The latter enzyme is responsible for transport of fatty acyl-CoA derivatives across the inner mitochondrial membrane.

2. Carnitine-palmitoyl transferase II subsequently liberates fatty acyl-CoA within the mitochondria. Fatty acyl-CoA undergoes β-oxidation, forming acetyl-CoA. Carnitine returns to the extra-mitochondrial space.

3. Acetyl CoA can then be completely oxidised in the tricarboxylic (Krebs) acid cycle, utilised in lipid synthesis or partially oxidised to ketone bodies.

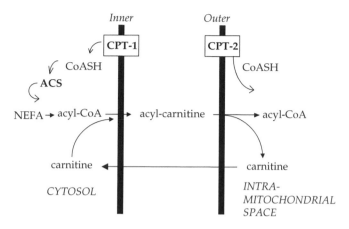

CPT-1 and 2 = carnitine–palmitoyl transferase
ACS = acyl-coenzyme A synthase
NEFA = non-esterified fatty acid
Acyl-CoA = acyl-coenzyme A
CoASH = coenzyme A
Modified with permission from Frayn KN. *Metabolic regulation.* 2nd ed.
Oxford, Blackwell Publishing, 2003.

Figure 1.2 Fatty acid transport across the mitochondrial membrane

Acetoacetate is in equilibrium with 3-hydroxybutyrate, the balance being dictated by the hepatic redox state. In ketoacidosis the plasma ratio of 3-hydroxybutyrate to acetoacetate ratio is typically elevated to about 3 : 1.

$$\text{acetoacetate} + NADH + H^+ \xrightarrow[\text{dehydrogenase}]{\text{3-hydroxybutyrate}} + NAD$$

Acetone is formed by the spontaneous decarboxylation of aceto-acetate:

$$\text{acetoacetate} \rightarrow \text{acetone} + CO_2$$

Elevated acetone concentrations in ketoacidosis do not contribute to the metabolic acidosis. Acetone is highly fat soluble and is slowly excreted through the lungs.

Ketone body disposal

With the exception of the liver, which lacks 3-oxo-acid CoA transferase, most tissues have the capacity to utilise ketone bodies. During treatment of ketoacidosis, oxidation of ketone anions gradually neutralises the acidosis through the generation of equimolar quantities of bicarbonate ions. Ketone body excretion via the kidney and lung are important modes of elimination in ketoacidosis.

Fluid and electrolyte depletion

Dehydration and electrolyte losses are prominent features of diabetic ketoacidosis.

- *Water.* When the renal threshold for glucose re-absorption in the proximal convoluted tubule is exceeded, the resulting osmotic diuresis leads to dehydration and secondary losses of electrolytes (Table 1.1). Ketonuria compounds the loss of both water and electrolytes.

- *Sodium.* Insulin deficiency and glucagon excess exacerbate sodium depletion via effects on renal sodium reabsorption. Hyperventilation, fever and sweating due to infection may

Table 1.1   Average deficits of electrolytes in adults with diabetic ketoacidosis

Sodium	500 mmol
Chloride	350 mmol
Potassium	300–1000 mmol
Calcium	50–100 mmol
Phosphate	50–100 mmol
Magnesium	25–50 mmol

further exacerbate fluid and electrolyte depletion, resulting in average losses of body water in adults of approximately 5 L. Increasing plasma osmolality leads to intracellular dehydration. Reduced renal blood flow resulting from extracellular dehydration impairs a major route of elimination of glucose and ketone bodies; adequate correction of dehydration is therefore important during the early phase of therapy.

- *Potassium.* Metabolic acidosis leads to displacement of intracellular potassium by hydrogen ions; these are subsequently lost in urine or vomit. Breakdown of cellular protein secondary to insulin deficiency compounds the loss of intracellular potassium. However, despite a considerable total body potassium deficit, serum potassium is usually normal or high at presentation of diabetic ketoacidosis. Acidosis, insulin deficiency and renal impairment all contribute to hyperkalaemia. Hypokalaemia at presentation signifies a marked deficiency of body potassium that in some patients may be enhanced by antecedent diuretic therapy.

- *Phosphate.* Total body phosphate deficiency is common in ketoacidosis and may be exacerbated by co-existing conditions such as chronic alcoholism. Insulin therapy stimulates cellular uptake of phosphate and a variable degree of hypophosphataemia is common during the treatment phase of diabetic ketoacidosis. Phosphate deficiency is associated with reduced red cell 2,3-diphosphoglycerate levels, resulting in reduced oxygen delivery to the tissues. However, the adverse effects on the oxyhaemoglobin dissociation curve are offset by the acidaemia of ketoacidosis (the Böhr effect). The benefits of phosphate supplements on the course and prognosis of diabetic ketoacidosis have not been substantiated in clinical trials. Large sample sizes are required to demonstrate statistically significant clinical benefits in diabetic ketoacidosis. Serum phosphate levels may be elevated despite a total body deficit. Some authorities recommend replacement of phosphate if levels fall below an arbitrary level, e.g. 0.5 mmol/L, although this is not common practice in the UK. A degree of caution is necessary as iatrogenic hypocalcaemia may complicate phosphate replacement.

- *Magnesium.* While the clinical significance of hypomagnesaemia that commonly accompanies diabetic ketoacidosis is also uncertain, it may exacerbate potassium deficiency.

The development of diabetic ketoacidosis is summarised in Figure 2.1.

Clinical features

The cardinal symptoms of ketoacidosis include

- rapidly increasing polyuria and polydipsia
- rapid weight loss – dehydration
- nausea and vomiting – hyperketonaemia is emetic
- generalised muscular weakness
- muscular cramps.

These are followed by serious signs of cerebral dysfunction:

- progressive drowsiness and obtundation
- coma.

While a decrease in the level of consciousness is common, coma is encountered in only about 10 per cent of patients. The mechanism by which ketoacidosis induces coma remains uncertain; impairment of consciousness correlates with plasma glucose concentration and osmolarity, coma at presentation being associated with a worse prognosis. Co-existing causes of coma such as stroke, head injury or drug overdose should be considered and excluded if

Table 1.2 Causes of impaired consciousness in patients with diabetes mellitus

- Diabetic ketoacidosis
- Hyperosmolar non-ketotic hyperglycaemia
- Hypoglycaemia
- Lactic acidosis
- Other causes:
  - Stroke (more common in diabetic patients)
  - Post-ictal (including hypoglycaemia – generalised tonic–clonic convulsions also cause a self-correcting lactic acidosis; see Chapter 6)
  - Cerebral trauma (may follow hypoglycaemia)
  - Ethanol intoxication (may induce or exacerbate hypoglycaemia in diabetic patients)
  - Drug overdose

serum osmolality is less than approximately 350 mOsmol/kg (Table 1.2).

Usually symptoms usually require several hours to develop, often following symptoms of an intercurrent illness. Physical signs are usually prominent in severe diabetic ketoacidosis.

- *Dehydration.* Variable; approximately 5 L in an average adult.

- *Hypotension.* Supine hypotension, in the absence of confounding effects of anti-hypertensive drugs, denotes more than 20 per cent depletion of extracellular fluid volume. Severe hypotension in ketoacidosis carries an adverse prognosis

- *Tachycardia.* Reflects dehydration, acidosis and sympathetic activation; drugs with anti-muscarinic effects, e.g. tricyclic antidepressants used for treatment of symptomatic neuropathy, may exacerbate tachycardia.

Severe diabetic ketoacidosis may develop within 24 hours.

Other clinical and biochemical features include the following.

- *Air hunger.* Acidosis stimulates the respiratory centre within the medulla oblongata, causing deep rapid respirations (Kussmaul breathing).

- *Ketotic fetor.* The odour of acetone may be obvious on the breath, although the capacity to detect acetone varies between individuals.

- *Hypothermia.* Another consequence of acidosis, which may mask a valuable sign of infection. Rectal temperature should be taken with a low reading thermometer if hypothermia is suspected; marked hypothermia carries an adverse prognosis.

- *Leukocytosis.* This is common with hyperketonaemia and does not necessarily indicate infection.

- *Gastroparesis.* A gastric succusion splash may be evident on abdominal examination as a consequence of gastric stasis; the stomach may become distended with several litres of contents, posing a risk of aspiration in patients with an impaired level of consciousness.

- *Abdominal pain.* Generalised abdominal pain may occur, particularly in younger patients with severe acidosis (see Chapter 2). If abdominal pain does not resolve with resolution of the acidosis, alternative causes should be suspected. Measurement of plasma amylase is unhelpful since levels may be raised non-specifically in ketoacidosis; ultrasound imaging of the pancreas may be of assistance in diagnosing pancreatitis.

Diagnosis

Delays in initiating therapy may have disastrous consequences. Diabetic ketoacidosis should be considered in any unconscious or hyperventilating patient. If there is any doubt about the severity of the metabolic disturbance in a diabetic patient with ketosis, the arterial pH should be measured. A brief clinical examination focuses on

• airway protection

• cardio-pulmonary status

• level of consciousness

• precipitating causes.

Bedside blood and urine tests should rapidly confirm the diagnosis. Treatment should then be commenced without delay. The initial clinical and biochemical assessment of a patient with suspected diabetic ketoacidosis is shown in Table 1.3.

• *Urine.* If available, should be tested for the presence of glucose and, most importantly, for ketones. The presence of protein, nitrites and leukocytes suggest infection.

• *Venous blood.* Minimum urgent laboratory investigations include measurement of

   ○ glucose (fluoride oxalate tube)

   ○ urea (blood urea nitrogen)

   ○ creatinine

   ○ sodium

   ○ potassium

   ○ full blood count with differential.

Some of the potential pitfalls in the diagnosis and management of diabetic ketoacidosis are summarised in Table 1.4.

Table 1.3 Initial assessment of patients with suspected diabetic ketoacidosis

Clinical history. Initially, brief and relevant (including previous episodes of ketoacidosis and potential precipitating causes).

Physical examination. Rapid but thorough assessment for signs of dehydration, level of consciousness, metabolic acidosis (Kussmaul respiration), hypotension, hypothermia, gastric stasis and any precipitating condition (e.g. pneumonia, pyelonephritis).

Biochemical assessment. Confirm diagnosis by bedside measurement of

- blood glucose (by glucose-oxidase reagent test strip)
- urine ketones ('Ketostix').

Venous blood is withdrawn for laboratory measurement of

- glucose
- urea (BUN)
- sodium
- potassium
- chloride (required for calculation of anion gap)
- ketones.

In addition take blood for

- full blood count
- blood cultures (in all cases)

Inspect plasma for turbidity (hyperlipidaemia).

Capillary or arterial blood gases (corrected for hypothermia) for

- pH
- bicarbonate
- pCO_2
- arterial pO_2.

Repeat laboratory measurement of blood glucose, electrolytes, urea, gases at 2 and 6 h.

Other investigations. Chest X-ray, culture of urine/sputum/faeces, electrocardiograph, sickle cell test etc., as indicated.

BUN = Blood urea nitrogen.

Table 1.4 Potential pitfalls in the diagnosis and management of diabetic ketoacidosis

---

• *Odour of acetone on the patient's breath.* a useful sign but many people cannot detect acetone

• *Fever.* may be absent in the presence of infection (peripheral vasodilatation causes cooling)

• *Blood leukocytosis.* neutrophil count may be non-specifically raised

• *Plasma sodium concentration.* may be falsely lowered initially by high lipid and glucose levels and may appear to rise suddenly after insulin treatment lowers plasma glucose and lipid levels

• *Plasma potassium concentration.* may be temporarily raised (by acidosis) despite severe total body potassium depletion

• *Plasma creatinine concentration.* may be falsely elevated (assay interference by ketone bodies)

• *'Ketostix' testing.* may show 'negative' or 'trace' result when lactic acidosis or alcoholic ketoacidosis coexist with diabetic ketacidosis (predominance of 3-hydroxybutyrate). Ketostix reaction may become temporarily stronger during treatment of diabetic ketoacidosis (conversion of 3-hydroxybutyrate to acetoacetate)

• *Plasma transaminases and creatine phosphokinase.* may be non-specifically raised

---

Practical points to consider include the following.

• *Glucose.* Hyperglycaemia is readily determined on capillary or venous blood using a glucose-oxidase reagent strip or blood gas analyser, pending confirmation by the clinical chemistry laboratory. Diabetic ketoacidosis presenting in the absence of marked hyperglycaemia is recognised but uncommon; absence of severe hyperglycaemia does not exclude ketoacidosis.

• *Ketones.* Plasma ketone body concentration should be measured (semi-quantitatively) with a nitroprusside-based reaction. These tests are essentially specific for acetoacetate and do not react with the principal ketoacid in diabetic ketoacidosis, i.e. 3-hydroxybutyrate; acetone reacts weakly. Experimental evidence in subjects with type 1 diabetes suggests that fasting results in ketoacidosis with smaller increments in blood glucose concentration compared with the non-fasting state. However, this should not be confused with mild starvation ketosis in the non-diabetic subject. In the absence of diabetes, serum glucose will be normal or slightly reduced by a severely reduced caloric intake for several days. The resulting mobilisation of fatty acids from adipocytes, a consequence of appropriately low insulin concentrations, leads to ketonuria. The brain gradually increases its utilisation of ketones as an alternative energy source and so severe ketosis does not develop. This physiological adaptation contrasts with the situation in diabetic ketoacidosis: the combination of hyperglycaemia with significant ketosis points to marked insulin deficiency.

> In starvation ketosis, serum glucose is in the low–normal range; the presence of ketosis with hyperglycaemia indicates severe insulin deficiency.

A severe metabolic acidosis in the absence of hyperglycaemia, or other obvious cause of acidosis such as renal failure, raises the possibility of alternative diagnoses.

1. *Alcoholic ketoacidosis.* This is encountered in chronic alcoholics, often following a binge, when carbohydrate intake is reduced due to intractable vomiting from gastritis or acute pancreatitis. Elevated circulating concentrations of counter-regulatory hormones resulting from dehydration and the consequences of acute alcohol withdrawal stimulate lipolysis and ketogenesis. Hepatic metabolism of alcohol induces a more reduced mitochondrial redox state; this increases the ratio of serum 3-hydroxybutyrate to acetoacetate to as high as 7–10 : 1, compared with 3 : 1 in diabetic ketoacidosis. Under these circumstances a negative or minor urine or plasma ketone reaction may give a misleading impression of the degree of the ketonaemia. Since hyperglycaemia is usually absent, treatment of acute alcoholic ketoacidosis comprises rehydration

Table 1.5   Causes of anion gap acidosis

Ketoacidosis
  Diabetic ketoacidosis
  Alcoholic ketoacidosis
Lactic acidosis
Chronic renal failure
Drug toxicity
  Methanol (metabolised to formic acid)
  Ethylene glycol (metabolised to oxalic acid)
  Salicylate poisoning

with intravenous dextrose and electrolyte replacement. This condition may be under-diagnosed.

2. *Lactic acidosis.* A similar diagnostic caveat may occasionally be encountered when significant lactic acidosis co-exists with ketoacidosis (see Chapter 6). Causes of an anion gap acidosis are shown in Table 1.5. The anion gap is elevated when serum

$$Na^+ - ([Cl^-] + [HCO_3]) > 10 \text{ mmol/L}$$

Potassium is not included in the calculation since the plasma level of this ion may be altered significantly by acid–base disturbances. The normal anion gap of approximately 10 mmol/L is accounted for by proteins, phosphate, sulphate and lactate ions. When the anion gap is increased, measurement of the plasma concentration of specific anions, e.g. ketone bodies, lactate, may confirm the aetiology of the acidosis. Although diabetic ketoacidosis usually presents as an anion gap acidosis, typically 25–35 mmol/L, a variety of acid–base disturbances have been reported.

- *Sodium.* Despite a proportionally greater loss of body water, plasma sodium concentrations are usually normal or low, although plasma electrolyte concentrations may be falsely depressed by grossly elevated plasma lipid concentrations in diabetic ketoacidosis. Plasma should therefore be inspected for turbidity.

Eruptive xanthomata and lipaemia retinalis are recognised complications that usually respond rapidly to treatment of the ketoacidosis.

- *Creatinine.* If measured using a colorimetric method, the serum creatinine concentration may be falsely elevated due to assay interference by acetoacetate; this may lead to an erroneous diagnosis of renal failure. Measurements in most modern laboratories will not be affected.

- *Enzymes.* Serum transaminases and creatine phosphokinase may be non-specifically elevated in diabetic ketoacidosis and may be mistaken for evidence of acute myocardial infarction.

- *Arterial blood gases.* The acidosis is quantified by measurement of pH, pCO_2 and bicarbonate concentration. Some gas analysers measure lactate, glucose and electrolytes.

- *Other tests.* Bacteriological culture of urine, sputum and blood is mandatory; broad-spectrum antibiotics should be administered promptly if infection is suspected. Testing for sickle cell and glucose-6-phosphate dehydrogenase deficiency may be indicated in selected patients.

Treatment

Investigations should not delay the initiation of treatment or transfer to a high-dependency or intensive care unit.

Aims of therapy

Treatment comprises rehydration with intravenous fluids, the administration of insulin and replacement of electrolytes. The treatment of ketoacidosis in children in considered in Chapter 2. The importance of general medical care and close supervision by trained medical and nursing staff deserves emphasis. A treatment flow-chart should be used (see Chapter 3) and updated meticulously. Accurate recording of fluid balance may necessitate a urinary catheter if no urine is passed in the first 4 h or so. An initial treatment plan for diabetic ketoacidosis in adults is shown in Table 1.6.

Table 1.6 Guide to treatment of diabetic ketoacidosis

Fluids and electrolytes

Volumes

- 1 L/h × 2–3, thereafter adjusted according to requirements

Fluids

- isotonic saline (0.9%) generally
- Hypotonic (0.45%) if serum sodium exceeds 150 mmol/L (no more than 1–2 L – consider 5% dextrose with increased insulin if marked hypernatraemia)
- 5% dextrose 1 L every 4–6 h when blood glucose has fallen to ≤15 mmol/L (severely dehydrated patients may require simultaneous saline infusion)

Sodium bicarbonate

- ~700 mL of 1.26% or 100 mL of 8.4% (if large vein cannulated) if pH < 7.0 (with extra potassium)

Potassium

- No potassium in first 1 L of fluid unless initial plasma potassium < 3.5 mmol/L
- Thereafter, add dosages below to each 1 L of fluid. If plasma K^+
  - <3.5 mmol/L, add 40 mmol KCl (severe hypokalaemia may require more aggressive KCl replacement)
  - 3.5–5.5. mmol/L, add 20 mmol KCl
  - >5.5 mmol/L, add no KCl.

Insulin

Continuous intravenous infusion

- 5–10 U/h (average 6 U/h) initially until blood glucose has fallen to ≤15 mmol/L. Thereafter, adjust rate (1–4 U/h usually) during dextrose infusion

(continues overleaf)

Table 1.6 (*continued*)

to maintain blood glucose ~6–11 mmol/L until patient is eating again.
Measure, and record, capillary glucose hourly.

- Capillary blood glucose (mmol/L)
- 0–3.9*
- 4–6.9
- 7–9.9
- 10–14.9

- Soluble insulin infusion rate
- 0   see note below*
- 1   unit per hour
- 2   units per hour
- 3   units per hour

Other measures

- Search for and treat precipitating cause, e.g. infection.

- Hypotension usually responds to adequate fluid replacement.

- Central venous pressure monitoring in elderly patients or if cardiac disease present.

- Pass nasogastric tube – with airway protection – if conscious level impaired.

- Pass urinary catheter if conscious level impaired or no urine passed within 4 h of start of therapy.

- Continuous electrocardiographic monitoring may warn of hyper- or hypokalaemia (potassium should be measured at 0, 2 and 6 h – and more often if indicated by levels outside target range).

- Adult respiratory distress syndrome – mechanical ventilation (100% O_2, postive pressure ventilation); avoid fluid overload.

- Mannitol (up to 1 g/kg intravenously) if cerebral oedema suspected. Parenteral dexamethasone as alternative; N.B. induces insulin resistance. Consider cranial CT scan to exclude alternative pathology (e.g. cerebral haemorrhage, venous sinus thrombosis).

- Treat thrombo-embolic complications if they occur.

- Meticulous clinical and biochemical record using a purpose-designed flow-chart.

*Note: Intravenous insulin should not be interrupted if at all possible. However, errors leading to significant hypoglycaemia, e.g. inadvertent interruption of i.v. dextrose, may necessitate temporary cessation of insulin while corrective action is taken, e.g. increasing the dextrose infusion rate and/or bolus of 20–30 mL of 50% dextrose into a large vein if symptomatic (see Chapter 4). Aim to restart i.v. insulin within 15–30 min, at a reduced rate if indicated, and/or with a higher rate of dextrose infusion; consider 10% dextrose. Since interruption of i.v. insulin risks relapse of ketoacidosis, some clinicians advocate continuing insulin at a reduced rate while correcting lesser degrees of hypoglycaemia with i.v. dextrose. Careful monitoring with attention to infusion apparatus and hourly checks on the volumes infused will help to minimise the risk of hypoglycaemia.

Correction of fluid and electrolyte depletion

- *Rehydration.* Adequate rehydration is an important aspect of treatment that contributes directly to reductions in hyperglycaemia and counter-regulatory hormone levels. Considerable variation in fluid and electrolyte disturbances are observed between patients and the following recommendations represent only a guide to therapy.

  ○ Rehydration is commenced with isotonic (0.9 per cent, containing 150 mmol each of Na^+ and Cl^-) saline containing appropriate potassium supplements (see below). Isotonic saline is used in preference to hypotonic saline – unless plasma osmolarity is significantly raised – in order to minimise the rapid movement of extracellular water into cells as blood glucose and osmolarity fall with treatment; such shifts have been implicated in the pathogenesis of the serious complication of cerebral oedema, discussed below. Rehydration of the patient must take account of continuing polyuria and approximately 6–10 L of fluid may be required during the first 24 h.

  ○ In an average adult, 1 L of saline is infused every hour for the first two to three hours. The rate of infusion is then adjusted according to the clinical state of the patient. Care is required in elderly patients or those with cardiac disease; monitoring of central venous pressure or pulmonary wedge pressure is recommended in these circumstances.

  ○ Occasionally, patients with relatively low admission plasma glucose concentrations may require a simultaneous infusion of dextrose to allow administration of sufficient insulin to suppress lipolysis and ketogenesis without inducing hypoglycaemia.

  ○ A rising serum sodium concentration (above 150 mmol/L) may necessitate the temporary substitution of hypotonic saline (75 mmol/L each of Na^+ and Cl^-) or even 5 per cent dextrose (with an appropriate increase in the dose of insulin if dextrose is used).

o When plasma glucose has fallen to $\leq$15 mmol/L, saline is discontinued and replaced immediately by 5 per cent dextrose, usually at a rate of around 250 mL/h. Undue delay in commencing dextrose infusion at this point may result in hypoglycaemia. Intravenous dextrose is given without interruption until the patient is eating again, since intravenous insulin must be continued (albeit usually at a lower dose – see below).

o Although the use of hypertonic (10 per cent) dextrose at this stage of treatment produces a slightly faster fall in total ketone bodies, this is not reflected in a more rapid resolution of the acidosis.

• *Potassium replacement.* Cardiac arrhythmias induced by iatrogenic hypokalaemia represent a major and avoidable cause of death. Hypokalaemia may also induce life-threatening weakness of respiratory muscles. Potassium is predominantly (98 per cent) an intracellular ion. Insulin treatment and rising pH stimulate the entry of extracellular potassium into cells.

o On average 20 mmol of potassium (administered as 1.5 g potassium chloride) will be required in each litre of fluid following the start of insulin therapy. Continuous electrocardiographic monitoring may indicate signs of hyper- or hypokalaemia, but plasma potassium concentration should be checked regularly (2 hourly at first) and potassium supplements adjusted appropriately.

o Particular care must be exercised in patients with renal failure, anuria or oliguria (less than 40 mL/h).

o If hypokalaemia is present (plasma potassium < 3.5 mmol/L) potassium supplements should be doubled to 40 mmol/h; if hyperkalaemia develops potassium should be temporarily halted, pending the result of further measurements.

Insulin therapy

The successive aims of insulin treatment in ketoacidosis are

- inhibition of lipolysis and hence ketogenesis
- suppression of hepatic glucose production
- enhanced disposal of glucose and ketone bodies by peripheral tissues.

Soluble (unmodified) insulin only has a plasma half-life of approximately 5 min, so intermittent i.v. injections lead to unpredictable and fluctuating plasma insulin concentrations. Maximal stimulation of potassium transport into cells occurs with pharmacological plasma insulin concentrations and the risk of hypokalaemia is therefore greater with large doses of insulin. With modern insulin regimens, complications of treatment such as hypokalaemia and late hypoglycaemia are less common than with the obsolete high-dose intermittent bolus regimens.

- *Intravenous insulin.* Soluble insulin is administered as a continuous intravenous infusion at a rate of 5–10 (usually 6) U/h. This produces steady plasma insulin concentrations in the high physiological (or pharmacological at the higher rates) range that adequately suppress lipolysis, ketogenesis and hepatic glucose production, even in the presence of elevated levels of catabolic hormones. Insulin is diluted to a convenient concentration (usually 1 U/mL) with isotonic saline in a 50 mL syringe and delivered by a syringe-driver infusion pump connected via a Y connector. The infusion apparatus should be flushed through before connection to the patient. Alternatively, insulin can be added to a 500 mL bag of isotonic saline and mixed gently; the insulin must be injected using a needle of sufficient length to clear the injection port of the bag.

- *Monitoring response.* Capillary blood glucose is checked at the bedside at hourly intervals and the infusion rate is reduced to 1–3 U/h, when blood glucose has fallen to ≤15 mmol/L. The infusion rate should be adjusted to maintain euglycaemia until the patient is eating again and subcutaneous insulin is recommenced (Table 1.6). The rate required at this stage will vary according to (1) the degree of insulin resistance (see above) and (2) the rate of dextrose infusion. Intravenous insulin at 6 U/h should produce a steady and predictable fall in plasma glucose concentrations, averaging 4–6 mmol/h in adults. The commonest causes of failure to respond are mechanical, i.e. problems such as the pump being inadvertently switched off or set at the wrong rate and blockage of the delivery line. It is sound practice to cross-check (and record on the flow-chart) the prescribed rate of insulin delivery against the volume infused each hour during treatment. During treatment of ketoacidosis there is conversion of 3-hydroxybutyrate to acetoacetate. Nitroprusside-based tests may therefore give the mistaken impression that ketosis is either not resolving or is worsening. A rising plasma bicarbonate will allay such fears.

- *Transfer to subcutaneous insulin.* The first subcutaneous injection should comprise or include a dose of short- or rapid-acting insulin. This should be administered 60 min before the i.v. insulin infusion is terminated to allow time for absorption of insulin from the subcutaneous depot.

Bicarbonate therapy

The role of bicarbonate in the management of diabetic ketoacidosis remains controversial. No large clinical trials in severely acidotic patients with diabetic ketoacidosis have been performed. However, blood pH levels < 7.0 may lead to life-threatening cardio-respiratory complications. Small doses of bicarbonate (approximately 100 mmol) may be beneficial if the patient is severely acidotic or if cardio-respiratory collapse appears imminent. However, it is possible that administration of bicarbonate into the extracellular space may actually exacerbate intracellular acidosis. Bicarbonate ions (which cannot diffuse across cell membranes) combine with H^+ ions extra-cellularly, producing carbonic acid, which dissociates into water and CO_2. The latter readily enters cells, where the reverse reaction occurs, generating H^+ (and bicarbonate ions) intracellularly. The solution of 8.4 per cent sodium bicarbonate is hypertonic and extremely irritant and should only be infused into a large (ideally central) vein; extravasated solution often causes extensive local necrosis. Bicarbonate should therefore be infused as an isotonic solution, i.e. $\sim$700 mL of 1.26 per cent solution (12.6 g, each litre containing 150 mmol each of Na^+ and HCO_3^-) given over 30 min and repeated if necessary to raise the pH to 7.0–7.2. Other reservations about the use of bicarbonate include the following.

- *Hypokalaemia.* This may be exploited in the treatment of severe hyperkalaemia. Otherwise, extra potassium (20 mmol potassium per 100 mmol bicarbonate) should be administered when bicarbonate is infused and plasma potassium concentration should be re-checked shortly afterwards.

- *Paradoxical acidosis of cerebrospinal fluid.* The clinical significance of this complication is uncertain.

- *Tissue hypoxia.* Bicarbonate may have adverse effects on the oxyhaemoglobin dissociation curve.

- *Overshoot alkalosis.* Complete correction of the acidosis should not be the objective, since concurrent metabolism of ketone anions may lead to over-alkalinisation.

- *Acceleration of ketogenesis.* In a controlled clinical study, the fall in ketone body and lactate concentrations was delayed in patients with diabetic ketoacidosis who received 150 mmol of sodium bicarbonate compared with saline.

- *Cerebral oedema.* Treatment with bicarbonate has also been linked with the development of cerebral oedema in children with diabetic ketoacidosis (see Chapter 2).

Complications of diabetic ketoacidosis in adults

Aspiration

The stomach of a patient with diabetic ketoacidosis may contain 1–2 L of fluid, and where consciousness is impaired there is a possibility of vomiting with inhalation of gastric contents. Nausea or vomiting in a patient who is semi-conscious should lead to insertion of a naso-gastric tube under controlled conditions, i.e. with intubation if necessary.

Adult respiratory distress syndrome

Adult respiratory distress syndrome has been reported occasionally in patients with ketoacidosis, usually in patients under 50 years. Clinical features include dyspnoea, tachypnoea, central cyanosis and non-specific chest signs. Arterial hypoxia is characteristic and chest radiography reveals bilateral pulmonary infiltrates. Management involves respiratory support with intermittent positive pressure ventilation and avoidance of fluid overload.

Thromboembolism

Thromboembolic complications are important causes of mortality in patients with hyperglycaemic emergencies arising as a consequence of dehydration, increased blood viscosity and increased coaguability. Disseminated intravascular coagulation has also been reported as a rare complication of diabetic ketoacidosis. The role of prophylactic anticoagulation has not been clearly established and routine anticoagulation is not recommended in view of the risks of haemorrhage. Clinically evident thromboembolism is treated conventionally.

Rhinocerebral mucormycosis

This aggressive opportunistic fungal infections occasionally develops in patients with diabetic ketoacidosis or other metabolic acidoses. The lesion arises in the paransal sinuses and rapidly invades adjacent tissues (nose, sinuses, orbit and brain). Treatment comprises correction of acidosis, wide surgical excision of affected tissue condition and parenteral anti-mycotic agents. The course is often fulminant; the condition carries a high mortality.

Further reading

Adrogue HJ, Wilson H, Boyd AE *et al.* Plasma acid–base patterns in diabetic ketoacidosis. *N Engl J Med* 1982; **307**: 1603–1610.

Alberti KGMM. Low-dose insulin in the treatment of diabetic ketoacidosis. *Arch Intern Med* 1977; **137**: 1367–1376.

Barrett EJ, DeFronzo RA, Bevilacqua S and Ferrannini E. Insulin resistance in diabetic ketoacidosis. *Diabetes* 1982; **31**: 923–928.

Kitabchi AE, Umpierrez GE, Murphy MB, Barrett EJ, Kreisberg RA, Malone JI *et al.* Management of hyperglycemic crises in patients with diabetes. *Diabetes Care* 2001; **24**(1): 131–153.

Kraut JA and Kurtz I. Use of base in the treatment of severe acidemic states. *Am J Kid Dis* 2001; **38**: 703–727.

Krentz AJ and Nattrass M. Acute metabolic complications of diabetes. In: Pickup JC, Williams G (Eds). *Textbook of Diabetes*, 3rd ed. Oxford. Blackwell 2003 pp. 32.1–24.

McGarry JD and Foster DW. Regulation of hepatic fatty acid oxidation and ketone body production. *Annu Rev Biochem* 1980; **49**: 395–420.

Miles JM, Rizza RA, Haymond MW and Gerich JE. Effects of acute insulin deficiency on glucose and ketone body turnover in man. *Diabetes* 1980; **29**: 926–930.

Nattrass M and Hale PJ. Clinical aspects of diabetic ketoacidosis. In: Nattrass M, Santiago JV (Eds). *Recent Advances in Diabetes*, 1st ed. Edinburgh. Churchill Livingstone 1984 pp. 231–238.

Schade DS, Eaton RP, Alberti KGMM and Johnston DG. *Diabetic Coma, Ketoacidotic and Hyperosmolar.* Albuquerque, NM. University of New Mexico Press 1981.

2

Diabetic Ketoacidosis in Childhood

Julie A Edge and David B Dunger

Summary

Approximately 25 per cent of children present in diabetic ketoacidosis at diagnosis of type 1 diabetes, and this remains a life-threatening condition.

Guidelines for treatment are necessary, although they must always be tailored to the individual. Resuscitation is the primary objective. This includes prevention of aspiration of gastric contents using a nasogastric tube and adequate – but not excessive – replacement of circulating volume.

Further management comprises replacement of fluids with 0.9 per cent saline, replacement of potassium losses and the institution of insulin using a continuous intravenous infusion.

Recovery is usually straightforward, but there is still a significant mortality and morbidity, largely arising from the unpredictable

Emergencies in Diabetes   Edited by Andrew J. Krentz
© 2004 John Wiley & Sons, Ltd   ISBN 0-471-49814-9

complication of cerebral oedema. The pathophysiology of this devastating condition is still unknown, and there is an ongoing debate as to whether it is related to the treatment received. It is prudent to ensure that changes in osmolality do not occur too quickly, and that rehydration is not excessive. However, until the cause of cerebral oedema is known, no guidelines can be considered completely infallible. Close supervision from senior members of staff is essential, and there should be early concern if progress is not as predicted.

Early assessment of the best place to nurse the child should be made, and clear instructions given to nursing staff for frequent monitoring of vital signs and neurological observations. Headache and behaviour change should be reported at any time to medical staff. Rapid intervention with intravenous mannitol and immediate transfer to an intensive care unit for assisted hyperventilation and additional support is necessary if signs of cerebral oedema develop.

Introduction

Diabetic ketoacidosis in childhood remains a serious and life-threatening condition despite improvements in the management of the fluid and electrolyte disturbances over the last few decades. Although increased awareness among primary health care teams should have led to earlier diagnosis, around a quarter of children still present in diabetic ketoacidosis at the diagnosis of type 1 diabetes; the proportion is even higher in very young children in whom diabetes is not recognised early. Forty per cent of children diagnosed under 4 years of age in an Oxford Regional cohort in 1990 had ketoacidosis at diagnosis and in 25 per cent it was severe, i.e. arterial pH < 7.1. After the initial diagnosis of type 1 diabetes, admission rates with diabetic ketoacidosis during childhood are around 0.2 per patient year. Episodes are usually associated with intercurrent illness. In the older child, insulin omission and psychological disturbance may result in recurrent hospital admissions.

Sadly, ketoacidosis is still the major cause of death in children with type 1 diabetes. Approximately one per cent of episodes among children may be complicated by cerebral oedema, which is the major cause of type 1 diabetes-related death in children under the age of 12 years. Ketoacidosis is the most common cause of death outside hospital in teenagers and young adults with type 1 diabetes.

> Diabetic ketoacidosis is the leading cause of death among children with type 1 diabetes.

Definition

As for adults, the definition of diabetic ketoacidosis is arbitrary. In practice, the term refers to decompensated type 1 diabetes resulting in hyperglycaemia, and a metabolic acidosis attributable to hyperketonaemia. Blood glucose is generally raised, but in some three per cent of cases it may be less than 15 mmol/L.

Pathophysiology

As discussed in Chapter 1, the primary cause of ketoacidosis is an absolute or relative insulin deficiency. Briefly, the effects of insulin deficiency and thus an increase in glucagon/insulin ratio in the portal circulation together with increases in levels of counter-regulatory hormones (catecholamines, cortisol and growth hormone) are summarised in Figure 2.1. Elevated levels of ketone bodies result from mobilisation of fatty acids from adipose tissues and their preferential β-oxidation within the hepatic mitochondria; the finite capacity of peripheral tissues to utilise ketone bodies

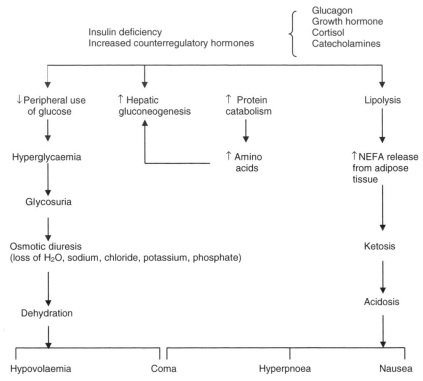

Figure 2.1 Schema of the pathophysiology of diabetic ketoacidosis. Adapted with permission from Lyen KR, Hale D, Baker L. Endocrine emergencies. In: Fleisher G, Ludwig S (Eds). *Textbook of Pediatric Emergency Medicine*. Baltimore, MD: Williams and Wilkins © 1983. NEFA = non-esterified fatty acids

contributes to the hyperketonaemia. Most of the acidaemia in diabetic ketoacidosis is accounted for by the production and dissociation of organic ketoacids, but lactic acidosis from tissue hypoperfusion may also contribute (see Chapter 6).

The regulation of ketosis during childhood differs in some respects from that observed in adults. In normal children, circulating levels of ketone bodies are relatively high prior to puberty. The finding of intermittent ketonuria is not unusual in non-diabetic young children, particularly after an overnight fast. During puberty, as plasma insulin levels increase, fasting ketone levels tend to fall. However, in adolescents with type1 diabetes, even when blood glucose levels are maintained at 5 mmol/L overnight using an intravenous insulin infusion, there is still a substantial increase in nocturnal ketogenesis, which appears to be due mainly to excessive growth hormone secretion. This may help explain the rapid decompensation that can occur in teenagers overnight following either a short episode of vomiting or the omission of bedtime insulin. Teenage girls in particular may present with severe acidosis despite only modest elevations of blood glucose.

Children develop ketosis more rapidly than adults.

Diabetic ketoacidosis is associated with severe losses of body fluids. The water deficit is made up of varying combinations from the osmotic diuresis, vomiting, hyperventilation and, when present, pyrexia. Sodium losses are also variable, depending on the predominating route of fluid loss, the duration of polyuria and the adequacy of renal perfusion. There is always total body depletion of potassium and phosphate, even though plasma levels of these ions may be low, normal or high. There will also usually have been some attempt by the child or its parent to correct the fluid losses with increased oral consumption of fluids, which can affect the blood biochemistry at presentation. Much of the information concerning the specific fluid and electrolyte deficits in diabetic ketoacidosis has been obtained from experiments carried out in adults in the 1930s, studies that have not been repeated in children. Thus there is little direct information concerning electrolyte and fluid losses in children; this may explain some of the historical debate concerning optimal management.

Differential diagnosis

The diagnosis is rarely difficult except in younger children, where the acidotic breathing pattern may easily be confused with an

Table 2.1 Differential diagnosis of diabetic ketoacidosis in children

Glycosuria/hyperglycaemia	Acidosis predominant
Physical stress, e.g. intercurrent infection with transient hyperglycaemia	Alcoholic ketoacidosis
MODY	Severe sepsis
Renal tubular defects	Certain inborn errors of metabolism
Corticosteroid treatment; N.B. may precipitate metabolic decompensation Hyperosmolar non-ketotic coma Type 2 diabetes	

MODY = maturity onset diabetes of the young.

upper or lower respiratory tract infection. In a small child, the characteristic smell of ketones on the breath may be attributed to fasting, but the diagnosis of diabetic ketoacidosis must be considered in any sick child, as the consequences of missing the diagnosis can be devastating. Further differential diagnoses are considered in Table 2.1.

Hyperosmolar non-ketotic hyperglycaemic coma (see Chapter 3) is rare in children; serum osmolality usually exceeds 300 mOsmol/L and ketosis is absent. The mechanism is likely to be prolonged dehydration with relative insulin sufficiency; it is more common in children with mental impairment. The management is similar to that of diabetic ketoacidosis, except that it has been recommended that insulin and fluids are given more slowly to prevent too rapid a fall in blood glucose and plasma osmolality.

Maturity onset diabetes of the young (MODY) is inherited in an autosomal dominant fashion and does not usually present with major metabolic decompensation. Insulin treatment is not usually required but may be necessary during intercurrent illness. The diagnosis should be firmly established using clinical and genetic criteria before any decision is made to discontinue insulin therapy. This also applies to the increasingly common situation wherein type 2 diabetes is diagnosed in childhood or adolescence.

Management

Diabetic ketoacidosis can be a rapidly changing condition, particularly in small children. Junior medical staff should routinely discuss such children with senior colleagues and should feel adequately supervised while undertaking treatment. Guidelines that are easy to understand and to use should be readily available in the hospital emergency department and on the wards, including high-dependency and intensive care units. The basic principles of management are as follows:

- correct the fluid losses

- reverse the acidosis and ketosis

- prevent complications such as aspiration of gastric contents, hypokalaemia, and cerebral oedema.

The guidelines that follow are based on those of the British Society for Paediatric Endocrinology and Diabetes (BSPED). These can be found in full on the BSPED website (www.bspe.shef.ac.uk), and a short algorithm version on the Diabetes UK website (www. diabetes.org.uk). These are very similar to the guidelines of the International Society for Paediatric and Adolescent diabetes (ISPAD; www.ispad.org). All of these are general guidelines for management. Note that treatment may need to be varied to suit the individual patient. Guidelines do not remove the need for frequent detailed reassessments of the individual child's progress. These guidelines are intended for the management of the following children:

- more than five per cent dehydrated

- and/or vomiting

- and/or drowsy

- and/or clinically acidotic.

Children who are five per cent dehydrated or less and not clinically unwell usually tolerate oral rehydration and subcutaneous insulin. Discuss this with the senior doctor on call.

Resuscitation (ABC)

Airway and breathing

The first priority in the treatment of diabetic ketoacidosis, as in the treatment of any life-threatening illness, is to protect and maintain the airway. If the childs level of consciousness is impaired, a nasogastric tube should be inserted immediately, aspirated and left on free drainage. An oral airway may also be necessary. If respiration is depressed, or there is accompanying respiratory pathology, intubation and ventilation may be required; if in doubt, this is the safest option. Tissue perfusion may be poor and, at least until the first arterial blood gas results are known, supplemental oxygen is generally administered by facemask.

Circulation

The next priority is to restore the circulating blood volume. However, true shock (hypotension and tachycardia) is very rarely present, and the degree of intravascular dehydration is often over-estimated. If there is truly reduced circulating volume, give 10 mL/kg 0.9 per cent saline over 10 min. This can be repeated to a maximum of 20–30 mL/kg at this stage, titrated against changes in tissue perfusion, or in the most severe cases against central venous pressure.

Clinical assessment

The clinical features of diabetic ketoacidosis are shown in Table 2.2.

Table 2.2 Clinical features of diabetic ketoacidosis in children

Symptoms	Signs
Polyuria	Lethargy
Thirst, polydipsia	Dehydration
Rapid weight loss	Blood pressure normal, rarely low
Abdominal pain	Kussmaul respiration, or later depressed
Weakness	Smell of ketones on breath
Vomiting	Temperature normal
Air hunger	20% disordered consciousness
Confusion, coma	10% unconscious

1. During the resuscitation phase a rapid clinical assessment should have been made of the following.

- *Airway, breathing and circulation.* See above.

- *Conscious level.* If the conscious level is impaired, or there is any change in neurological status during treatment, the Glasgow Coma Score should be serially recorded, and deteriorating conscious level treated as an emergency (see section on cerebral oedema below).

- *Degree of dehydration.* It has recently been recognised that the degree of dehydration in children is often over-estimated by clinical methods, and that signs such as loss of skin turgor or elasticity occur at around three per cent dehydration, and not at five per cent as is often quoted. Capillary refill time, tested by applying digital pressure, may be a useful technique for the assessment of dehydration in small children, as long as they are not exposed to a cold environment.

- *Weight of child.* This is crucial to the fluid management, therefore every effort should be made to weigh the child. If this is not possible because of the clinical condition, use the most recent clinic weight as a guideline, or an estimated weight from centile charts.

2. Full clinical assessment can be deferred until the child has been resuscitated. Attending doctors and nurses should be aware of the following.

- Abdominal pain is a frequent accompaniment of diabetic ketoacidosis in children; a surgical emergency should not be assumed until a period of rehydration and insulin and electrolyte replacement has been allowed.

- Pyrexia is not a feature of uncomplicated ketoacidosis, and a source of infection should be sought if it is present.

Laboratory assessment

Hyperglycaemia can be confirmed quickly by a high capillary blood glucose measurement, but it is important to ensure that reagent strips are fresh, that reflectance meters are well maintained and that staff are trained in their use. Ketone measurements are also possible on capillary blood, or urine if available. Treatment can then be started while the results of further tests, such as plasma electrolytes, are awaited. Suggested laboratory investigations are listed in Table 2.3. Arterial or capillary blood should ideally be used for acid–base assessment to confirm the acidosis, but where the facilities are not available venous pH and bicarbonate may be reasonable substitutes. Subsequently, acid–base status can be monitored using venous or non-arterialised capillary blood gases, since, although these will show a slightly higher CO_2 and bicarbonate, and slightly lower pH, the differences are not usually clinically significant.

Table 2.3 Suggested laboratory investigations in diabetic ketoacidosis

Investigation	Notes
Venous plasma glucose	• To confirm capillary result
Sodium, potassium, chloride, phosphate, calcium	• There may be artefactual lowering of sodium due to hyperlipidaemia
	• Chloride will help to define type of acidosis particularly during treatment
Plasma urea (BUN), creatinine	• Creatinine may be falsely elevated by hyperketonaemia; not usually a problem with modern chemical pathology laboratories
Blood gases, pH, bicarbonate	• If oxygen saturation is available, a venous or capillary sample is sufficiently accurate, otherwise use arterial sample
Urinary ketones	• Bedside blood ketone measurement may be helpful but insufficient evidence yet in children
FBC, PCV	• PCV may support clinical evidence of dehydration
	• Leucocytosis extremely common in ketoacidosis and does not necessarily imply infection
Urine culture	• If clinically indicated
Blood culture, CXR, throat swab	• Only if clinically indicated
Plasma amylase	• If abdominal pain severe and continues after adequate initial treatment

FBC = full blood count; PCV = packed cell volume; CXR = chest X-ray; BUN = blood urea nitrogen.

Instructions for nursing staff

A decision should be made at an early stage as to where the child should be nursed. If the child is very young, comatose or shocked, or if ward staff are exceptionally busy or inexperienced, then admission to an intensive care unit would be appropriate. Urinary catheterisation may be helpful in the comatose larger child but is not generally recommended.

Ensure full instructions are given to the *senior* nursing staff, emphasising the need for

- strict fluid balance of input and output, including oral fluids and weighing of nappies

- urine testing of *every* sample for ketones (may be superceded by bedside blood ketone measurements in some centres)

- hourly capillary blood glucose measurements

- hourly or more frequent neurological observations initially

- reporting *immediately* to the medical staff, even during the night, symptoms of *headache* or any change in either conscious level or behaviour, since these might indicate the development of cerebral oedema

- reporting any changes in the electrocardiograph trace, especially T wave changes

- recording body weight twice daily.

Fluids

1. *Choice of intravenous fluid.* After restoration of the circulating volume, the main residual fluid deficit is within the intracellular compartment. Historically, relatively hypotonic solutions were recommended, but a failure of plasma sodium concentration to rise during treatment has been linked with the development of cerebral oedema (see below). Most authors would therefore now recommend using isotonic (0.9 per cent) saline for the first few hours before changing to a more hypotonic solution, such as 0.45 per cent saline. 0.18 per cent saline is no longer

recommended. In practice, the fluid type is usually changed once the blood glucose concentration has fallen to around 10–15 mmol/L, but if this occurs very early during treatment, there is a possibility of giving too little sodium. In this situation, isotonic saline should be continued simultaneously with sufficient dextrose to avert hypoglycaemia during the latter stages of treatment. During such combination therapy, care should be taken to ensure that overall fluid volume is appropriate.

2. *Volume of fluid.* The volume of fluid to be replaced is based on the clinical assessment of the deficit plus maintenance fluid requirements, with the proviso that ongoing losses are also replaced. Clinical assessment of the degree of dehydration cannot be precise, and it is important not to over-estimate the degree of dehydration. The rate at which the fluids are given is an area of contention. It has been standard practice to give initial fluid rapidly initially, and then slow down the rate. However, since the rapid infusion of large volumes of fluid has been proposed as one risk factor for the development of cerebral oedema, once the circulating blood volume has been restored, it is reasonable to correct the remaining fluid deficit slowly and evenly over the next 24 or even 36 or 48 h. Furthermore, slow rehydration has been used successfully in adults with diabetic ketoacidosis and, paradoxically, it may lead to more rapid restoration of acid/base balance.

3. *Practicalities of fluid administration.*

- It is *essential* that *all* fluids administered are documented carefully, particularly the fluid that is given in the initial phase of therapy and during transfer to the ward; this is where most errors occur.

- By this stage, the circulating volume should have been restored. If not, give a further 10 mL/kg 0.9 per cent saline or 4.5 per cent albumin over 30 min.

- Otherwise, once circulating blood volume has been restored, calculate fluid requirements as follows:

requirement = maintenance + deficit

[deficit (litres) = % dehydration × body weight (kg)]

- To avoid over-zealous fluid replacement, which may be a risk factor for cerebral oedema, never assess dehydration as more than 10 per cent. Include the volume of fluid that may have been given during resuscitation.

Age	Maintenance values
0–2 yrs	80 mL/kg/24 h
3–5	70 mL/kg/24 h
6–9	60 mL/kg/24 h
10–14	50 mL/kg/24 h
adult (>15)	35 mL/kg/24 h

Add maintenance and deficit and give the total volume evenly over the next 24 hours. i.e.

$$\text{hourly rate} = \frac{\text{maintenance} + \text{deficit}}{24}$$

Example:
A 20 kg 6 year old boy who is 10 per cent dehydrated will require 10 per cent × 20 kg = 2000 mL deficit

plus   60 mL × 20 kg = *1200 mL* maintenance
                    = 3200 mL over 24 hours = 133 mL/h.

- It may be preferable (although there is no definite evidence) to lengthen the period of rehydration to 48 h in very young children or those who are very hyperosmolar with high plasma sodium levels or very high blood glucose levels. Discuss this with a senior clinician.

Insulin

- Although insulin resistance has been shown to be a feature of diabetic ketoacidosis, in practice large doses of insulin are not required. A continuous low-dose intravenous infusion of 0.1 U/kg/h of soluble (unmodified) insulin is an effective and simple method for reversing the metabolic acidosis, and is associated with a lower incidence of hypoglycaemia and hypokalaemia than higher doses. A bolus of insulin is not necessary as large doses may cause a rapid reduction in blood glucose which may be undesirable.

- There are some who believe that younger children (especially the under 5s) are particularly sensitive to insulin and therefore require a lower dose of 0.05 U/kg/hour. There is no evidence to support the lower dose, and only the larger dose has been shown to correct hyperglycaemia and reverse ketosis.

- Insulin should not be added to the replacement fluid bag, but should be infused using a separate syringe pump, so that adjustments to fluid and insulin can be made independently.

Potassium

- Potassium is mainly an intracellular ion, and there is always massive depletion of total body potassium in diabetic ketoacidosis, although initial plasma levels may be low, normal or even high. Circulating levels will *fall* once insulin therapy is commenced.

- Potassium replacement should therefore be started immediately unless anuria is suspected or there are peaked T waves on the electrocardiogram. The infusion should be altered according to subsequent plasma electrolyte results to maintain plasma potassium concentration within the normal range.

- Add 20 mmol potassium chloride (KCl) to every 500 mL bag of fluid if normokalaemia.

- A cardiac monitor should be observed frequently for T wave changes.

Bicarbonate

As discussed in Chapter 1, this is rarely, if ever, indicated. Profound acidosis can theoretically be a cause of poor myocardial contractility, although there is no evidence to support this in children. It has been our recent practice only to use bicarbonate at a blood pH of less than 6.9, or if there is evidence of poor circulation after adequate administration of resuscitation fluid. The commonest reason for the failure of acidosis to resolve is inadequate restoration of the circulating blood volume or late institution of insulin therapy, which therefore fails to suppress ketogenesis.

Phosphate

Diabetic ketoacidosis is associated with severe phosphate depletion due to excessive urinary losses, and once insulin treatment is started levels will fall, because phosphate, like potassium, is taken up by the cells. Although plasma concentrations may fall in adults to levels known to have been associated with impaired cardiac function, respiratory failure and reduced red cell 2,3-diphosphoglycerate concentrations, these complications are rarely seen, and have not been reported in children. There is no evidence that replacement is beneficial; it may precipitate symptomatic hypocalcaemia.

Subsequent management

- Check plasma urea and electrolytes 2 h after resuscitation has begun and then at least 4 hourly during treatment.

- Check fluid balance and the clinical state of the child at least 4 hourly, to ensure that positive fluid balance is maintained.

- If a massive diuresis continues fluid input may need to be increased; measurement of urinary electrolytes may be helpful to determine the type of fluid replacement required. If large volumes of gastric contents are aspirated, these should be replaced with 0.45 per cent saline containing 10 mmol/L KCl.

• If acidosis is not resolving in the first few hours, resuscitation may have been inadequate; therefore, consider giving more saline. Sepsis is another possibility that should be considered.

• With initial resuscitation, the blood glucose often falls rapidly. A fall of more than 5 mmol/L/h has been implicated in the development of cerebral oedema, although no case–control studies support this link. However, if it falls rapidly halve the insulin infusion rate and/or increase the concentration of dextrose in the replacement fluid.

• Once the blood glucose has fallen steadily to 10–15 mmol/L, fluid replacement should continue with a glucose-containing solution, usually 5 per cent dextrose. This permits continuing intravenous insulin therapy whilst avoiding iatrogenic hypoglycaemia.

• Subsequently, blood glucose should be maintained by adjusting the dextrose infusion rather than reducing the insulin infusion rate lower than 0.05 U/kg/h, since both insulin and glucose are required for the reversal of ketogenesis and glycogenolysis; rapid relapse may ensue if insulin is interrupted.

• Once the child is rehydrated, and is tolerating food and fluids, subcutaneous insulin can be substituted for intravenous insulin. The first dose of subcutaneous insulin should be given an hour before terminating the intravenous insulin infusion; this avoids transient insulinopenia. Note that urinary ketones may be detectable for one or two days, owing to the conversion of β-hydroxybutyrate (which is not measured by conventional urine sticks) to acetoacetate. However, there may still be a degree of insulin resistance at this stage, so larger doses of insulin than usual may be required to suppress ketogenesis.

Table 2.4   Complications of diabetic ketoacidosis

Under-treatment:	
Unresolved acidosis	• Try further fluid resuscitation, increase insulin dose, consider sepsis
Blood glucose not falling	• Increase insulin dose; ensure adequate hydration
Recurrence of ketoacidosis	• Restart protocol from beginning
Over-treatment:	
Unrecognised hypokalaemia	• Regular electrolyte measurements and ECG monitoring
Hypoglycaemia	• Reduce but *do not stop* insulin, increase dextrose concentration in fluids
Others:	
Aspiration of gastric contents	• Early nasogastric intubation will prevent this
Cerebral oedema	• Aetiology not understood
Pulmonary oedema/adult respiratory distress syndrome	• Commoner in adults

ECG = electrocardiograph.

Complications

These are listed in Table 2.4. With meticulous management and observations, severe hypokalaemia or hypoglycaemia and aspiration pneumonia are now uncommon, and the greatest risk is from cerebral oedema.

Cerebral oedema

This is almost exclusively a condition of childhood; over 95 per cent of cases in the largest reported series occurred under the age of 20 years, with one-third under the age of 5 years. Mortality from cerebral oedema is around 25–30 per cent and around 30 per cent of survivors are left with major neurological morbidity. It is more common in children with newly diagnosed type 1 diabetes.

Table 2.5 Clinical features of cerebral oedema complicating diabetic ketoacidosis

- headache
- confusion
- irritability
- reduced conscious level
- convulsions
- small pupils
- increasing blood pressure, slowing pulse
- papilloedema – not always present acutely
- possibly impaired respiratory drive

Subclinical brain swelling appears to be common during the treatment of diabetic ketoacidosis, and may be present even before intravenous rehydration is commenced. Whether severe, sudden clinical cerebral oedema is an extension of this process, or whether the two are distinct entities, remains to be determined. The clinical signs of cerebral oedema are variable. Most cases have occurred between 4 and 12 hours from the start of treatment. Signs and symptoms of cerebral oedema are presented in Table 2.5.

Cerebral oedema is a feared complication of diabetic keto-acidosis in children.

If warning features are not recognised, there is commonly a sudden deterioration, manifest as loss of consciousness, appearance of fixed dilated pupils or respiratory arrest. Possible contributing factors include

- cerebral anoxia from the reduced blood volume and haemo-concentration

- high initial plasma glucose concentration

- excessive rates of intravenous fluid administration

- a rapid fall in plasma sodium concentration.

Animal studies have suggested that insulin is required for cerebral oedema to occur, and hypoxia resulting from rapid bicarbonate infusion has also been implicated. However, none of these theories provides a complete explanation, and the fact that the incidence has remained the same over several decades, despite changes in fluid regimens, suggests that the fluid regimen may not be a crucial factor. More recent studies suggest that the most severely dehydrated children are at greatest risk.

> The aetiology and optimal treatment of cerebral oedema complicating diabetic ketoacidosis remain uncertain.

Only half of patients have a period of neurological deterioration during which intervention might be effective before respiratory arrest. Therefore, prevention of this complication remains one of the most important goals of the management of diabetic ketoacidosis in children. If cerebral oedema is suspected

- exclude hypoglycaemia

- inform senior medical staff immediately

- give intravenous mannitol 0.5 g/kg stat (= 2.5 mL/kg mannitol 20 per cent over 15 min); administer *as soon as possible*

- restrict intravenous fluids to two-third maintenance requirements and replace deficit over 72 rather than 24 h

- transfer child to intensive care unit

- if necessary arrange for the child to be intubated and hyperventilated to reduce blood pCO_2

- exclude other diagnoses by computed tomography – other intracerebral events may occur (thrombosis, haemorrhage or infarction) and present in the same way

- intracerebral pressure monitoring may be indicated

- repeated doses of mannitol (dose as above every 6 h) can be used to control intracranial pressure (recently it has been suggested that hypertonic saline may be a more effective osmotic agent, but insufficient studies have yet been performed).

Further reading

Edge JA. Cerebral oedema: are we any nearer finding a cause? *Diabetes Metab Res Rev* 2000; **16**: 316–324.

Edge JA, Ford-Adams ME and Dunger DB. Causes of death in children with insulin dependent diabetes 1990–96. *Arch Dis Child* 1991; **81**: 318–323.

Glaser N, Barnett P, McCaslin I, Nelson D, Trainor J, Louie J, Kaufman F, Quayle K, Roback M, Malley R and Kuppermann N. Risk factors for cerebral oedema in children with diabetic ketoacidosis. *N Engl J Med* 2001; **344**: 264–269.

Krane EJ, Rockoff MA, Wallman JK and Wolfsdorf JI. Subclinical brain swelling in children during treatment of diabetic ketoacidosis. *N Engl J Med* 1985; **312**: 1147–1151.

Pinkney JH, Bingley PJ, Sawtell PA, Dunger DB and Gale EAM. Presentation and progress of childhood diabetes mellitus: a prospective population-based study. *Diabetologia* 1994; **37**: 70–74.

Sperling MA. Diabetic ketoacidosis. *Pediatr Clin N Am* 1984; **31**(3): 591–610.

3

Hyperosmolar Non-ketotic Hyperglycaemia

Hans J Woerle and **John E Gerich**

Summary

Hyperosmolar non-ketotic hyperglycaemia is one of the most serious endocrine emergencies. Prompt and adequate therapy is critical. Outcome depends on early correction of fluid deficit and treatment of the underlying precipitating illness. Any middle aged or elderly person with signs of mental status deterioration and severe dehydration must be suspected of hyperosmolar non-ketotic hyperglycaemia.

Diagnosis. Plasma glucose > 30 mmol/L with plasma osmolarity > 320 mOsm/kg. Severe dehydration with pre-renal uraemia is the rule. Note lack of ketoacidosis (pH > 7.3; plasma bicarbonate > 15 mmol/L); cf. diabetic ketoacidosis.

Emergencies in Diabetes   Edited by Andrew J. Krentz
© 2004 John Wiley & Sons, Ltd   ISBN 0-471-49814-9

Therapy. Fluid replacement (0.9 per cent saline 1–2 L over the initial 1 h) aiming for gradual restoration of normal osmolarity (6–12 L over next 12 h). Control hyperglycemia using i.v. insulin 5–10 U/h in adults until plasma glucose has fallen to ~15 mmol/L when insulin infusion rate is reduced to 1–4 U/h. Prevention of hypokalaemia typically requires 20–40 mmol potassium chloride per litre, depending on renal function. General medical support and treatment of precipitating factors, e.g. infection, are important; patients often have serious comorbidity.

Acute complications. These include thrombo-embolic episodes, rhabdomyolysis, seizures and transient focal neurological signs.

Mortality. The case fatality rate is high – up to 50 per cent depending on co-existing conditions.

Long-term management. A proportion of patients do not require insulin long term. Avoid precipitating factors in the future wherever possible.

Pathogenesis

Hyperosmolar non-ketotic hyperglycaemia is a serious and life threatening condition that carries an average mortality rate of ~15 per cent, mortality is increased in the presence of concomitant illnesses and advancing age to over 50 per cent. The syndrome is not uncommon, being generally responsible for approximately 1:1000 hospital admissions, more so in patients over the age of 60 years. Hyperosmolar non-ketotic hyperglycaemia is characterised by

- severe hyperglycemia

- dehydration with pre-renal uraemia

- hyperosmolarity.

Table 3.1 Common precipitating factors for the development of hyperosmolar non-ketotic hyperglycemia

Acute illness	Drug therapy
Infection (30–60%)	Corticosteroids
(most commonly cellulitis,	Diuretics
pulmonary and urinary tract)	Phenytoin
Sepsis	Chlorpromazine
Stroke	Cimetidine
Renal failure	Diazoxide
Heat stroke	β-adrenergic blockers
Hypothermia	Antipsychotics – typical and
	atypical
Pancreatitis	Immunosuppressive agents
Severe thermal burns	
Endocrine diseases:	
• type 2 diabetes	
• acromegaly	
• cushing's syndrome	
• thyrotoxicosis	

Precipitating factors include conditions or medications leading to severe dehydration and impaired insulin secretion and/or insulin resistance. The most common are summarised in Table 3.1. The most frequent and important precipitating factors are those that cause dehydration. The stress of acute illnesses, e.g. acute infections, is usually accompanied by insulin resistance manifested by increased secretion of hormones that antagonise the actions of insulin, e.g. glucagon, catecholamines, cortisol and growth hormone together with certain cytokines, which impair insulin sensitivity and insulin secretion (see Chapter 1). Some conditions (e.g. acute pancreatitis) and medications (e.g. phenytoin, diazoxide) directly reduce insulin secretion, while others induce insulin resistance (e.g. anti-inflammatory doses of corticosteroids).

Hyperosmolar non-ketotic hyperglycaemia generally develops over several days to weeks. Fever, vomiting and polyuria without appropriate fluid intake, as may occur frequently in elderly people, lead to severe dehydration. Approximately 80 per cent of affected patients have been previously diagnosed with type 2 diabetes or impaired glucose tolerance. Dehydration and hyperosmolarity promote insulin resistance and impair insulin secretion. Since β-cell function is already impaired in patients with type 2 diabetes and impaired glucose tolerance, an adequate increase in insulin secretion does not occur; severe hyperglycaemia develops. An osmotic diuresis due to hyperglycaemia in combination with inadequate fluid intake leads to a further fluid loss and decreased renal perfusion. Ultimately a vicious circle is formed in which glucose enters plasma much faster than it can be taken up by tissues or excreted by the kidneys.

> Hyperosmolar non-ketotic hyperglycaemia develops gradually over hours or days.

The typical patient is elderly with a plasma glucose level above 30 mmol/L, plasma hyperosmolarity greater than 320 mOsm/Kg and a body water deficit of 20–25 per cent, i.e. approximately 10 L. This water loss causes an increased plasma tonicity, which shifts water together with potassium out of cells into the extracellular space. At the same time, hydrogen ions are shifted into the cell. Consequently, despite marked renal potassium losses, plasma potassium levels are usually normal or elevated, and the blood pH is in the normal range at time of admission.

> Dehydration is a prominent features of hyperosmolar non-ketotic hyperglycaemia.

Up to 70 per cent of patients present with frank coma, which may be solely the result of severe dehydration and hyperosmolarity. The remaining patients show mild to moderate signs of lethargy; partial seizures and other focal, reversible neurological deficits are well recognised. A minor degree of ketosis or hyperlactataemia may be present, the latter reflecting inadequate tissue perfusion (see Chapter 6). However, by definition plasma ketone body levels, and levels of their precursors – non-esterified fatty acids, are much lower than those seen in diabetic ketoacidosis; accordingly, the arterial pH is generally above 7.3. Since diabetic ketoacidosis is also a state of hyperosmolarity, several authors have suggested that hyperosmolar non-ketotic hyperglycaemia should not be differentiated from diabetic ketoacidosis, but rather be recognised as being at one end of the spectrum of severe acute metabolic derangements in diabetes. It has been proposed that a major pathophysiological differentiation is maintainence of a degree of endogenous insulin secretion in hyperosmolar non-ketotic hyperglycaemia, in contrast to the severe relative or absolute insulin deficiency in diabetic ketoacidosis.

- *Endogenous insulin secretion.* It is suggested that in the hyperosmolar non-ketotic hyperglycaemia syndrome the presence of circulating insulin is sufficient to suppress lipolysis and thus prevent ketosis (see Chapter 1); however, the residual function of the β-cells may not be enough to prevent hyperglycaemia. There is, however, surprisingly little evidence to support this hypothesis. In fact, the only two studies comparing plasma insulin concentrations in diabetic ketoacidosis and hyperosmolar non-ketotic hyperglycaemia did not find any significant difference in plasma insulin concentrations, at least in the peripheral circulation.

- *Hyperosmolality.* Another theory is that dehydration–hyperosmolarity and hyperglycaemia play the major role in the absence of ketoacidosis in this condition: hyperosmolarity, hyperglycaemia and dehydration reduce lipolysis (and thus availability of the main precursor availability for ketogenesis, i.e. fatty acids) and directly impair hepatic ketogenesis and insulin secretion.

- *Counter-regulatory hormone levels.* In addition, patients with hyperosmolar non-ketotic hyperglycaemia generally have lower plasma cortisol and growth hormone levels, which would provide less stimulation of lipolysis. Regardless of the pathophysiological mechanism, from a clinical point of view the distinction between hyperosmolar non-ketotic hyperglycaemia and diabetic ketoacidosis is of little importance since the main elements of therapy for both conditions, i.e. fluid replacement and insulin, are similar. In general, however, patients with hyperosmolar non-ketotic hyperglycaemia require more fluids and less insulin.

Significant ketosis and acidosis are not features of hyperosmolar non-ketotic hyperglycaemia.

Diagnosis

Hyperosmolar non-ketotic hyperglycaemia is a medical emergency that requires a high degree of suspicion for prompt recognition and treatment; a fingerstick capillary glucose measurement will readily indicate the presence of marked hyperglycaemia. The diagnosis should be considered in any person who exhibits signs of

- dehydration
- abnormal mental status or focal neurological signs
- hypovolemia or shock.

Although usually regarded as a condition of the elderly, the syndrome has occasionally been reported in children. The first approach is a rapid but thorough history and physical examination with special attention to

- prior history of diabetes mellitus – hyperosmolar non-ketotic hyperglycaemia may be the initial manifestation of diabetes

- mental status

- signs of broncho-pulmonary infection

- airway, cardiovascular and renal status

- common precipitating conditions (Table 3.1).

Coma may be present with severe hyperosmolality, but levels less than $\sim$350 mOsm/kg should prompt consideration of alternative causes, e.g. stroke a sedative drug overdose. Typically, conscious patients report increasing polydipsia and polyuria and progressive weight loss from dehydration for several days, sometimes accompanied by nausea and vomiting, the latter symptoms being more frequently encountered in diabetic ketoacidosis. Pre-existing renal impairment may result in more severe degrees of hyperglycaemia because renal losses are less pronounced; the degree of dehydration will be reduced. Occasionally abdominal pain may mimic symptoms of an acute abdomen although, once again, this is more often encountered in diabetic ketoacidosis, particularly in children (see Chapter 2). Since acute pancreatitis and other surgical conditions may precipitate hyperosmolar non-ketotic hyperglycaemia in predisposed individuals, an intra-abdominal cause should be excluded. Signs of dehydration include

- loss of skin turgor

- dry mucous membranes

- tachycardia

- hypotension

- oliguria.

Initial laboratory evaluation:

- venous plasma glucose (usually >30 mmol/L)
- plasma sodium (normal or increased)
- arterial blood pH (normal or slightly reduced)
- plasma osmolality (>320 mOsm/kg)
- plasma potassium (normal or increased)
- plasma creatinine and urea (increased)
- blood count with differential – leukocytes (increased).

Plasma sodium concentration is reduced due to movement of water from the intracellular to extracellular compartment consequent on hyperglycaemia-associated hyperosmolality. However, countering this effect, urinary sodium losses, if prolonged, may lead to marked hypernatraemia. The osmotic diuresis also leads to urinary losses of phosphate, calcium and magnesium. As for diabetic ketoacidosis, depletion of total body levels of these ions is not reflected in admission plasma concentrations. Additionally,

- bacterial cultures of blood, urine and sputum should be obtained if ongoing infection is suspected
- a chest radiograph should be obtained
- electrocardiography should be considered.

Treatment

As in the management of diabetic ketoacidosis (see Chapters 1 and 2), a flow sheet monitoring treatment given, responses to treatment and the results of serial laboratory determinations is extremely useful (Figure 3.1).

	Time Elapsed (h)
	Glucose
	Na
	K
	Cl
	CO_2
	Urea (BUN)
	Creatinine
	pH
	Serum osmolality
	Insulin given
	Fluids given
	Urine output
	Net fluid balance
	Mental status*
	BP
	Pulse
	Temp
	CVP

Laboratory

* N, normal; D, drowsy; S, stuporous; C, comatose.
Notes: BUN, blood urea nitrogen; CVP, central venous pressure; BP, blood pressure.
Glasgow coma scale is used widely in UK.

Figure 3.1   Flow sheet for monitoring treatment

• Management in an intensive care setting might be required, depending on the clinical condition of the patient and presence of co-morbidities. Therapy should be initiated without delay.

• Diligent monitoring of clinical and biochemical variables is required.

   ○ Capillary blood glucose is measured hourly at the bedside during the initial phase of treatment, i.e. until blood glucose is normalised and stable.

   ○ Serum electrolytes and fluid balance should be determined hourly at least for the first three hours and if satisfactory responses occur subsequently these can be measured at 2–3 h intervals.

   ○ Other responses to treatment, e.g. fluid balance, mental status, etc. should be assessed at similar intervals. It is recommended that the chest X-ray be repeated after 24 h of treatment because pulmonary infiltrates not present initially may become evident after rehydration.

By 12 h or so, appropriate correction of hyperglycemia and hyperosmolarity have usually been obtained and 60–80 per cent of the fluid deficit restored; subsequent correction of residual fluid deficits can be achieved orally since patients should be ready to resume eating and drinking at this point. Although treatment needs to be individualised, a generally applicable algorithm for adults is given in Figure 3.2.

Fluid replacement

Severe dehydration is the leading element in the development of hyperosmolar non-ketotic hyperglycaemia and is a major determinant

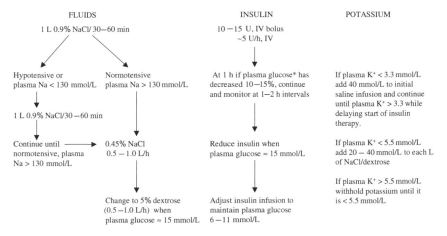

Figure 3.2   Suggested algorithm for the management of HNKH

of morbidity and mortality. Consequently, rapid and adequate fluid replacement is crucial. In all patients, an intravenous line should be placed, and fluid therapy should be initiated immediately to prevent avoidable complications due to dehydration (stroke, myocardial infarction, acute renal failure, etc.).

- Regardless of the initial plasma sodium concentration, it is recommended that 1 L of 0.9 per cent saline be infused during the initial 30 min. If the initial plasma potassium is below 3.5 mmol/L, add 40 mmol/L of saline and continue to add potassium until the plasma potassium is above 3.5 mmol/L (see below).

- If the patient is hypotensive or has a plasma sodium level below 130 mmol/L, another litre of 0.9 per cent saline should be infused over the next 30–60 min.

- Subsequently, and in the absence of hypotension, hydration may be continued with either 0.9 or 0.45 per cent sodium chloride. No data are available from randomised studies to guide selection of initial fluid replacement; the use of 0.9 per cent saline is widely accepted although some authorities recommend 0.45 per cent saline. During the first 2 h the average adult patient should receive 2–4 L of fluid. Thereafter the infusion rate can be reduced to 0.5–1.0 L/h depending on urinary volumes and cardiac status.

• The severity of dehydration may ultimately require up to 12–15 L within the first 12–24 h, taking continued diuresis into account. Some authorities recommend calculating fluid deficits. However, these consider only extracellular dehydration and have not been shown to be superior to clinical assessment.

> No controlled clinical studies are available to guide selection of crystalloids for rehydration.

A thorough attention to urine output, signs of fluid overload such as pulmonary congestion and jugular venous distension must guide the rate of fluid administration; early bladder catheterisation is helpful, although it should be removed promptly after recovery. Central venous pressure and continuous urine output should be monitored in patients with

• a history of congestive heart failure

• a history of renal insufficiency

• acute renal failure

> Accurate ascertainment of fluid balance is an important aspect of management.

Fluid repletion itself will have a major impact on lowering plasma glucose concentrations. Correction of volume contraction will enhance renal glucose excretion and reduce overactivity of the sympathetic nervous system, leading to enhanced hepatic and peripheral insulin sensitivity. Too rapid a fall of plasma glucose should be avoided to prevent dangerous fluid and electrolyte shifts. Fluid may shift too rapidly from extra- to intracellular space with the risk of cerebral oedema and compromised perfusion of the brain and other vital organs.

Insulin therapy

Insulin therapy is perhaps less important than fluid replacement and may be withheld – temporarily – until plasma potassium is above 3.5 mmol/L in the unusual situation when patients present with severe hypokalaemia.

- After an initial i.v. bolus (10–15 U), which some clinicians regard as optional, insulin should initially be infused at a low rate, i.e. 5–10 U/h – typically 6 U/h in an adult. Note that the short half-life of insulin in the circulation requires an uninterrupted intravenous infusion.

- The plasma glucose should not be lowered by more than 15 per cent per hour. When the plasma glucose reaches ≤15 mmol/L, an infusion of 5 per cent dextrose (plus potassium as necessary) should be started; 100–150 mL/h is usually appropriate. In most cases, dextrose will replace saline at this point; saline can be infused simultaneously if necessary. Since the objective is to maintain blood glucose on a plateau, the insulin infusion rate should be lowered and adjusted so as to gradually achieve values between approximately 5 and 10 mmol/L. This will usually be achieved at rate of 0.5–4 U/h, with concomitant infusion of dextrose.

If the plasma glucose initially fails to decrease, the volume replacement regimen should be reassessed and the integrity of the insulin infusion should be checked, e.g. was it made up correctly? Is it functioning correctly? etc.

Suggested infusion regimen

5 mL of U-100 human soluble insulin in 1 L of saline; at an infusion rate of 10 mL/h this delivers 5 U/h insulin. If plasma glucose has not decreased by 15 per cent within 2 h of insulin and volume replacement, the insulin infusion rate should be *doubled* and the response reassessed at hourly intervals.

Potassium replacement

- If the initial plasma potassium concentration is 3.5–5.5 mmol/L, co-administer 20 mmol potassium chloride per hour, added to the infusate, be it saline or dextrose. Adequate fluid and insulin administration will rapidly lower the plasma potassium as potassium re-enters the intracellular compartment.

- No potassium should be infused if hyperkalaemia (>5.5 mmol/L) is present. Care must be exercised in patients with pre-existing renal impairment or oliguria. Electrocardiographic monitoring is recommended in all patients receiving higher potassium doses for hypokalaemia, or showing any abnormal rhythm (including tachycardia).

Some clinicians recommend that one-third of the potassium might be given as potassium phosphate if plasma phosphate is low (i.e. <0.5 mmol/L), since phosphate shifts along with potassium back into the intracellular compartment. Potential complications of severe hypophosphataemia, i.e. <0.3 mmol/L, are

- haemolytic anaemia
- muscle weakness
- depressed systolic cardiac and respiratory performance.

On the other hand, controlled clinical trials have not demonstrated any benefit from routine phosphate therapy in diabetic ketoacidosis (see Chapter 1). It should also be borne in mind that excessive administration may cause hypocalcaemia with tetany, soft tissue calcification and renal failure. Therefore, care is required and it is prudent to monitor plasma phosphate levels in patients being given potassium phosphate. Most patients appear to recover fully without the need for intravenous phosphate replacement.

> The role of intravenous phosphate replacement in the treatment of hyperosmolar non-ketotic hyperglycaemia is uncertain.

Other aspects of management

After 2–4 h, when plasma glucose levels have decreased appreciably and several litres of fluid have been administered, it is crucial at this point to monitor the mental status of the patient. Any reversion of initial improvement may be a sign of too vigorous rehydration and/or too rapid reduction in plasma osmolarity, causing the development of pulmonary or, occasionally, cerebral oedema. The best evidence for an appropriate fluid management is a constant improvement in mental status. Furthermore, hourly glucose and electrolyte checks are recommended to avoid hypoglycaemia and hypokalaemia.

Complications

Thrombo-embolic complications

Despite the high frequency of thrombo-embolic complications in patients with the hyperosmolar syndrome, the role of prophylactic anticoagulation is unclear. Anti-coagulation in an acutely sick patient carries risks of gastrointestinal haemorrhage – an occasional cause of death. The alternative approach is to treat clinically overt thrombo-embolic events as they arise; this approach will lead to occasional failure to recognise the insidious development of serious thrombosis. The risk–benefit equation will differ between individual patients and this presents the clinician with a dilemma.

Rhabdomyolysis

Non-traumatic rhabdomyolysis in patients with greater degrees of hyperosmolarity occasionally precipitates acute renal failure. This complication has been associated with a poor prognosis in some reports. The diagnosis is suggested by a greatly elevated serum creatinine kinase concentration (usually >1000 IU/L) in the absence of alternative causes such as myocardial infarction, stroke or pre-existing end-stage renal failure.

Discharge planning

It is important to emphasise the need to continue some insulin to avoid relapses of hyperglycaemia and/or hyperosmolarity. Subcutaneous insulin treatment should not be initiated too early; insulin may be absorbed poorly and erratically from subcutaneous tissue before effective perfusion is re-established.

- By 12–24 h, once the patient is able to eat and drink, subcutaneous insulin can be commenced, either as a multiple-daily (basal–bolus) regimen or as twice-daily injections of biphasic insulin. Avoid using a sliding scale regimen for subcutaneous insulin; this treats hyperglycaemia after it occurs when the objective is to prevent hyperglycaemia.

- Approximately 0.5–1.0 U/kg/day will usually be needed, in divided doses: half is given as insulin glargine or isophane at bedtime and the remaining half as short-acting insulin before meals in proportion to the carbohydrate content, with somewhat more given with breakfast; start with an injection of soluble (or rapid-acting) insulin. Pre-prandial and bedtime blood glucose levels are measured to guide changes in insulin doses. In general, we do not recommended discontinuation of insulin for several days, if at all. Insulin requirements are still increased above what patients may require under normal life conditions due to acute insulin resistance.

• As insulin requirements decrease, other choices of therapy may be considered; the decision to withdraw insulin should be made by an experienced clinician.

A proportion of patients admitted with hyperosmolar non-ketotic hyperglycaemia will be able to discontinue insulin and maintain good glycaemic control with oral anti-diabetic agents or even dietary measures. Precipitating factors, e.g. drugs, should be avoided to prevent a recurrence.

Some patients with hyperosmolar non-ketotic hyperglycaemia are able to discontinue insulin therapy after recovery.

Further reading

American Diabetes Association. Hyperglycemic crisis in patients with diabetes mellitus. *Diabetes Care* 2003; **26**: S109–S117.

Fishbein HA and Palumbo PJ. Acute metabolic complications in diabetes. In: National Diabetes Data Group, ed. *Diabetes in America 1995* pp. 283–291. Bethesda, MD: National Institutes of Health.

Gerich JE. Hyperosmolar nonketotic coma. In: Kassirer J, ed. *Current Therapy in Internal Medicine,* 3rd ed. 1991 pp. 1278–1281. Philadelphia, PA: Decker.

Kitabchi AE, Umpierrez GE, Murphy MB, Barrett EJ, Kreisberg RA, Malone JI and Wall BM. Management of hyperglycemic crises in patients with diabetes. *Diabetes Care* 2001; **24**: 131–53.

Matz R. Hyperosmolar nonacidotic diabetes. In: Porte D Jr and Sherwin RS, eds. *Diabetes Mellitus: Theory and Practice,* 5th ed. 1997 pp. 845–860. Amsterdam: Elsevier.

4

Insulin-induced Hypoglycaemia

Simon R Heller

Summary

Hypoglycaemia may occur following ingestion of drugs such as aspirin or alcohol and in those who develop an insulinoma, but by far the commonest cause is insulin treatment in people with insulin-treated diabetes. Most episodes are due to the limitations of current subcutaneous insulin delivery, which is too crude to prevent inappropriately raised plasma insulin levels in between meals.

The brain is vulnerable to hypoglycaemia since cerebral tissue cannot store carbohydrate and needs a continuous glucose supply. Severe hypoglycaemia leads to impaired cognition, confusion and coma. Very low levels (<1 mmol/L) that are prolonged for hours can cause death or permanent cerebral damage.

While many patients experience multiple episodes without apparent ill effects, repeated severe hypoglycaemia may

Emergencies in Diabetes   Edited by Andrew J. Krentz
© 2004 John Wiley & Sons, Ltd   ISBN 0-471-49814-9

cause significant cognitive impairment. At diagnosis and for
some years after, patients with type 1 diabetes can mount a
powerful endocrine response to hypoglycaemia during which
glucagon and adrenaline resist the glucose-lowering effect of
insulin. Activation of the autonomic nervous system produces
symptoms that alert patients, giving them time to treat
themselves.

With increasing duration of either type 1 or type 2 diabetes,
both the hormonal and symptomatic responses to hypoglycaemia often become impaired, a change also observed during
intensive insulin therapy. This makes it more difficult for
patients to identify the onset of hypoglycaemia and, although
not a major problem if mild, poses a considerable risk to those
severely affected. It is caused in part by periods of hypoglycaemia, which cause maladaptive changes within the brain.

Recent work has shown that programmes of hypoglycaemia
avoidance can restore symptoms and awareness, at least in
part. The crucial issue in managing severe hypoglycaemia is to
reverse the threat of cerebral dysfunction and damage.

Intramuscular glucagon is the treatment of choice; its administration needs no expert training or equipment and can be
given rapidly by family members or paramedics. Intravenous
glucose is only needed in the few who fail to respond
to glucagon. Failure to recover conciousness after ~1 h is
indicative of possible cerebral damage; full recovery can follow
coma of some hours.

Epidemiology and frequency

Standard therapy with twice daily insulin leads to severe
hypoglycaemic episodes in around 10 per cent of patients with
type 1 diabetes per annum. This risk generally rises threefold
among those attempting tight glucose control with either multiple

daily injections or continuous subcutaneous insulin infusion. The risk of severe hypoglycaemia is considerably less in type 2 diabetes, affecting around 0.5 per cent in a year of those taking sulphonylureas (see Chapter 5) and 2–3 per cent in patients taking insulin. Nevertheless, since type 2 diabetes is ten times more prevalent, as many patients with insulin-treated type 2 experience a severe episode as those with type 1 diabetes.

> The risk of severe insulin-induced hypoglycaemia is considerably lower in patients with type 2 diabetes in comparison with patients with type 1 diabetes.

As the duration of type 2 diabetes increases, so the risk of severe hypoglycaemia rises. This is probably due to a combination of

- failing counter-regulatory responses (see below)

- symptomatic unawareness and an increasing dependence on the vagaries of exogenous insulin.

Vulnerability of the brain to hypoglycaemia

During prolonged starvation the brain utilises ketone bodies as alternative fuels and has also been shown to metabolise lactate. However, under normal conditions, the brain depends entirely upon glucose to sustain its metabolism. Unlike other tissues, the brain has only limited stores of carbohydrate such as glycogen, which can be rapidly converted to glucose. If the supply of glucose to the brain is reduced below a critical value for even a few minutes, then cerebral function becomes impaired. In humans, this occurs at a glucose concentration of just above 3 mmol/L and is initially manifest as a lengthening of reaction time, which can be measured experimentally. If blood glucose continues to fall cerebral function progressively deteriorates, leading to increasingly impaired cognition, confusion and eventually loss of consciousness. The glucose concentration at which these changes occur varies within and between individuals on different occasions. Some people with diabetes can sometimes appear to behave completely normally at a glucose concentration around 1 mmol/L; at other times the same blood glucose concentration will render the patient unconscious. The cause of this variability is unclear but perhaps relates to the ability of the brain to adapt to hypoglycaemia through mechanisms that maintain intra-neuronal glucose or via utilisation of alternative metabolic fuels (see above).

> Brain function is dependent on a continuous supply of glucose.

Morbidity and mortality

It is not possible to perform experimental studies in humans to establish the precise levels of hypoglycaemia that produce permanent brain injury. Animal experiments have shown that at glucose levels of below 1 mmol/L the electroencephalogram tracing becomes flat; if sustained this causes severe and permanent brain damage. However, under certain circumstances, the human brain may withstand even this level of glucose without permanent effects.

- In the 1940s and 1950s, severe insulin-induced hypoglycaemia was used to treat severe psychiatric conditions such as schizophrenia. Although it was eventually shown to be an ineffective treatment, some patients were subjected to repeated episodes of insulin shock at glucose levels well below 1 mmol/L. These produced coma and seizures, and although some patients died or were left with permanent brain damage others apparently suffered surprisingly few permanent effects.

- Severe hypoglycaemia (blood glucose below 1 mmol/L) of longer duration, i.e. hours, can cause permanent brain injury. On other occasions, however, even short-lived episodes can also result in sustained cognitive impairment.

- Nonetheless, severe episodes of hypoglycaemia caused by accidental or suicidal overdose of insulin do not inevitably lead to irreversible brain damage. When patients recover consciousness they often exhibit severe memory loss, which then recovers over the following weeks or months. Even prolonged coma lasting 1–2 days can be followed by complete recovery.

> Severe, recurrent or prolonged hypoglycaemia may cause permanent brain damage.

Cerebral damage secondary to hypoglycaemia seems to be a relatively rare cause of death in diabetic patients treated with insulin; however, insulin-induced death may result from other mechanisms. In a seminal paper, Tattersall and Gill (1991) investigated all unexpected sudden deaths in patients with type 1 diabetes in the UK under the age of 40 during a single year. They identified only two deaths that could be attributed to hypoglycaemic brain damage with certainty. This study highlighted the cases of 22 young people who were found dead in an undisturbed bed. There was strong circumstantial evidence implicating hypoglycaemia; many of the 22 had been experiencing intermittent nocturnal hypoglycaemia in the months before their death. Tattersall and Gill speculated that a cardiac arrhythmia might have been involved. Recent studies have shown that experimental hypoglycaemia in humans causes lengthening of the electrocardiographic QT interval, a known cause of fatal dysrhythmias in some other conditions. These conduction defects appear to be caused by a combination of falls in plasma potassium, secondary to

- sympatho-adrenal activation

- direct effects of circulating adrenaline on the myocardium.

What remains unclear is whether certain individuals with diabetes are particularly vulnerable to QT lengthening during hypoglycaemia. Since pharmacological selective β-adrenergic blockade prevents these changes, if it proves possible to identify those most vulnerable to QT lengthening then they might be protected by the use of such agents; this hypothesis remains to be tested.

> The dead-in-bed syndrome in patients with type 1 diabetes is thought to be a result of severe nocturnal hypoglycaemia.

Why is hypoglycaemia common in diabetes?

Unphysiological insulin delivery

Insulin treatment is designed to mimic the physiology of the islet β-cell, delivering substantial and precise amounts of insulin to cover the hyperglycaemia that follows meals, yet ensuring much lower but stable basal concentrations in between. However, current subcutaneous insulin preparations are inadequate to this task even when administered in multiple small doses. The use of rapid-acting insulin analogues delivered via continuous subcutaneous infusion using an external electromechanical pump perhaps provides the closest approximation to physiological insulin replacement. However, even this form of insulin delivery produces inadequate insulin concentrations during meals and inappropriately raised plasma insulin concentrations when absorption from the gastrointestinal tract is complete. This leads to a combination of

- high post-prandial glucose concentrations

- vulnerability to hypoglycaemia between meals. This is a particular problem at night when a period of >12 h can separate the evening meal and the breakfast that follows the morning after. Even if patients take a bedtime snack they remain susceptible to nocturnal hypoglycaemia during the second half of the night.

> Current insulin regimens fall short of normal physiology, thereby presenting the risk of hypoglycaemia.

The limitations of intermittent subcutaneous insulin delivery arise partly because insulin enters the systemic rather than the portal circulation. The inability to deliver the insulin directly to the liver, as happens when insulin is secreted from the β-cells, causes higher insulin levels in the peripheral circulation. In addition, short-acting insulin preparations tend to self-associate into hexamers, delaying the rate of absorption of insulin into the bloodstream from subcutaneous depots. Different approaches have been tried to develop a basal insulin preparation, i.e. that mimics normal background low-level insulin secretion, that has stable and consistent characteristics. However, lente and isophane preparations not only produce an undesirable peak of insulin but have considerable inter- and intra-subject variability.

Recently introduced rapid-acting and so-called basal insulin analogues have improved pharmacokinetics that may prove more useful than conventional insulin preparations. To date, clinical trial data indicate that these novel analogues provide a relatively modest albeit useful advance with reduced rates of hypoglycaemia at similar levels of glycaemic control. Clinicians – and patients – need to gain more experience with these analogues in order to determine their optimal application. As for conventional insulin, the particular circumstances of the patient will require careful individualisation of therapy to attain glycaemic targets safely.

> Insulin analogues with improved pharmacokinetic profiles are associated with a reduced risk of hypoglycaemia.

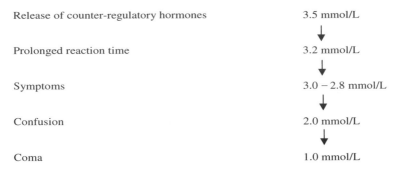

Release of counter-regulatory hormones	3.5 mmol/L
Prolonged reaction time	3.2 mmol/L
Symptoms	3.0 − 2.8 mmol/L
Confusion	2.0 mmol/L
Coma	1.0 mmol/L

Figure 4.1   Sequence of events during hypoglycaemia

Pathophysiology of hypoglycaemia in diabetes

Recovery from insulin-induced hypoglycaemia would take many hours if dissipation of insulin were the sole mechanism (Figure 4.1). Additional physiological mechanisms help to resist the glucose lowering effect of insulin and restore blood glucose after an episode of hypoglycaemia. Secretion of counter-regulatory hormones

- promotes glucose release from the liver

- opposes glucose uptake in peripheral tissues such as fat and muscle.

The most important of these hormones, in terms of recovery from hypoglycaemia, are glucagon and adrenaline, although others such as growth hormone and cortisol make a minor contribution (Table 4.1). These are precisely the same hormones that, when present in excess in

Table 4.1   Counter-regulatory hormones

*Glucagon
*Adrenaline
Cortisol
Growth hormone

*Major effects on recovery from acute hypoglycaemia

concert with insulin deficiency, promote major metabolic decompensation such as diabetic ketoacidosis (see Chapter 1).

- *Glucagon.* This hormone ranks high in the hierarchy of hormonal defences against hypoglycaemia, causing a prompt and substantial release of glucose from the liver. However, within a few years of diagnosis of type 1 diabetes the glucagon response to hypoglycaemia becomes progressively impaired. While the cause of this maladaptation remains unknown, increasing evidence suggests that β-cell destruction prevents the appropriate fall in local insulin concentration within the islet, which stimulates the α-cells to release glucagon. As the glucagon response fails, patients with diabetes become increasingly dependent upon the release of adrenaline to help to restore circulating glucose concentrations.

- *Adrenaline.* Release of adrenaline reflects activation of the sympatho-adrenal system, which generates a set of characteristic symptoms that alert patients to a falling plasma glucose concentration. Some individuals, particularly those with diabetes of long duration, also fail to release adrenaline during hypoglycaemia; this combined hormonal failure leads to a major increase in the risk of hypoglycaemia. As described below, this occurs because

1. those affected not only lack the hormonal mechanisms to raise blood glucose,

2. they can no longer reliably identify an impending episode of hypoglycaemia because warning symptoms are blunted or absent.

Symptoms of hypoglycaemia

Patients with insulin-treated diabetes rely on the physiological responses to hypoglycaemia to alert them to a falling glucose that

Table 4.2 Symptoms of hypoglycaemia

Neuroglycopenic	Autonomic
Confusion	Tremor
Irritability and bad temper	Sweating
Aggression	Palpitations
Lack of concentration	
Diminished conscious level	
Coma	

prompts them to take action by taking refined carbohydrate (Table 4.2). Symptoms are generated through a combination of

1. sympathoadrenal activation (often termed autonomic symptoms) and

2. cerebral dysfunction caused by a failing glucose supply to the brain (termed neuroglycopenic symptoms).

Each patient learns to recognise his or her own pattern of symptoms, although these can vary over time, even day to day.

- *Autonomic symptoms.* In the early years after diagnosis, autonomic symptoms are usually more prominent and patients have sufficient time to correct impending hypoglycaemia. However, those individuals who lose their sympatho-adrenal response note a reduction in autonomic symptoms such as sweating and tremor. Increasingly, the patient has to depend upon neuroglycopenic symptoms such as loss of concentration.

- *Neuroglycopenic symptoms.* These reflect deteriorating cerebral function, and so by the time these develop the cognitive ability of those affected is already diminished. Unless patients can take steps to raise their blood glucose within a few minutes any further decline will, through neuroglycopenia, render them incapable of responding appropriately; without prompt external assistance severe hypoglycaemia may result, leading to coma or convulsions.

Hypoglycaemia unawareness

Overall, around 25 per cent of patients with type 1 diabetes experience difficulties in identifying when their blood glucose concentration is low; this situation is probably the rule in those with diabetes of long duration. The majority of patients have some degree of unawareness after 20 years or more of diabetes. However, hypoglycaemia unawareness can become a major clinical problem for a few individuals with type 1 diabetes regardless of duration. This situation increases the risk of severe hypoglycaemia sevenfold and can devastate the lives of both the patient and their families. Those severely affected are unable to drive motor vehicles and many find that their jobs are impossible to hold down.

> Loss of the warning symptoms of hypoglycaemia – hypoglycaemia unawareness – increases the risk of severe recurrent hypoglycaemia.

As outlined above, symptomatic awareness of hypoglycaemia largely depends upon an intact sympatho-adrenal response; it is the failure of this response which causes the clinical problem of hypoglycaemia unawareness. Although a sympatho-adrenal response still occurs, it is only activated at a low glucose concentration, i.e. approximately 2.5 mmol/L, the normal level for activation being around 3.5 mmol/L. It is clearly hazardous for those affected to try to maintain blood glucose levels close to normal by embarking on intensive insulin therapy. Frequent blood glucose monitoring will reduce the risk of a severe episode of hypoglycaemia, but affected patients should be encouraged to keep their blood glucose levels slightly above normal. For many this proves a difficult prospect, as they are often more worried about the risks of long-term complications resulting from hyperglycaemia.

> Hypoglycaemia unawareness may be reversed with meticulous avoidance of low blood glucose concentrations.

Causes of hypoglycaemia in insulin-treated patients

The traditional causes include

- excessive insulin doses

- missed meals

- inappropriate physical exercise.

In blaming the patient, invoking these factors fails to recognise what is increasingly appreciated as the main issue, i.e. ineffective insulin delivery. Many severe episodes of hypoglycaemia have no discernible explanation and probably, at least in part, reflect the variability of absorption of conventional insulin preparations. Anyone with insulin-treated diabetes, even with relatively poor overall glycaemic control, is at risk of the occasional severe episode, particularly during the night. Unsurprisingly, attacks are more likely in those whose aim is to maintain blood glucose concentrations close to normal (Table 4.3). This is in part because of a greater probability of low blood glucose values in those striving for near normoglycaemia but also because recurrent hypoglycaemia itself induces a failure of the physiological defences that oppose hypoglycaemia.

Table 4.3 Factors associated with reduced awareness of hypoglycaemia and an increased risk of hypoglycaemia

- Duration of diabetes
- Intensive insulin therapy
- Drugs, including alcohol
- Extremes of age

Duration of diabetes

Increasing duration of disease leads to progressive failure of insulin secretion in both type 1 and type 2 diabetes. As patients become increasingly dependent on exogenous injected insulin, they develop more erratic plasma insulin profiles. This makes them prone to hypoglycaemic episodes, particularly during the night, where the use of insulin preparations such as isophane, which has a peak of action in the early hours, has its greatest effect. Both of the main hormonal defences against hypoglycaemia are compromised as a function of the duration of disease.

- As discussed above, diminishing endogenous insulin secretion probably contributes to a failure of the glucagon response.

- The failure of the sympatho-adrenal response to hypoglycaemia in some patients is also related to increasing disease duration, although its cause is unclear. The belief that it is due to classic autonomic neuropathy is probably incorrect since some patients with severe autonomic neuropathy on cardiovascular reflex testing can mount a brisk sympatho-adrenal response. Further-more, many individuals with impaired counter-regulatory responses have normal autonomic function tests.

Tight glycaemic control and the effects of antecedent hypoglycaemia

Intensive insulin therapy is now known to be an important cause of reduced physiological defences to hypoglycaemia and unaware-ness. Despite efforts to exclude high-risk patients, the incidence of severe hypoglycaemia was increased several-fold among patients randomised to the intensive treatment arm of the US Diabetes Control and Complications Trial compared with the conventional treatment group; the latter had a significantly higher mean glycated haemoglobin concentration.

The increased risk of hypoglycaemia appears to be due to periods of antecedent hypoglycaemia that usually accompanies intensification of treatment. The changes appear similar to those observed with increased disease duration with a resetting of the threshold for activation of the autonomic response and symptoms to a glucose level below rather than above that for cognitive dysfunction. The site and precise nature of the abnormality are unknown but presumably the cerebral pathways responsible for sensing and activating the autonomic response are disrupted. This might be due to adaptation to hypoglycaemia within the central nervous system or possibly modulation by one of the counter-regulatory hormones. Cortisol is known to have powerful effects on neuronal function and infusing cortisol to levels seen during hypoglycaemia can produce impaired hormonal responses and symptoms in response to subsequent episodes. Thus, recurrent hypoglycaemia can produce a vicious circle of reduced physiological protection leading to a greater risk of subsequent hypoglycaemia and eventually a state of hypoglycaemia unawareness.

Prior episodes of hypoglycaemia alter the glycaemic threshold for secretion of counter-regulatory hormones.

Since short-lived hypoglycaemic episodes can cause severe functional defects without any apparent structural change, it follows that avoidance of hypoglycaemia might reverse the defect. This has now been demonstrated in clinical studies in which meticulous avoidance of hypoglycaemia led to recovery of both symptoms and the hormonal response to hypoglycaemia. In these studies it was possible to restore awareness of hypoglycaemia, at least in part, without significantly worsening blood glucose control, although HbA_{1c} concentration tended to rise. Furthermore, hypoglycaemia reversal programmes, although requiring intensive input from diabetes health care professionals, is within the scope of most diabetes units, particularly as those severely affected are relatively rare. The essential principle is avoidance of any hypoglycaemia, however mild, through a combination of frequent self-monitoring of blood glucose by the patient allied to a willingness to accept less stringent glucose targets.

Alcohol

Alcohol, while not directly lowering blood glucose, prevents recovery from hypoglycaemia via inhibition of hepatic gluconeogenesis. This results from the altered redox state generated by the metabolism of ethanol. Alcohol can therefore turn a mild hypoglycaemic attack into a severe and prolonged episode. It also suppresses some of the symptoms of hypoglycaemia such as tremor and this, combined with impaired cognition, can induce a temporary state of hypoglycaemia unawareness. The danger of unrecognised hypoglycaemia is increased by the similarity of symptoms of hypoglycaemia to intoxication with alcohol. Thus, friends and relatives may assume that a patient exhibiting odd behaviour due to hypoglycaemia is drunk and leave them to sleep it off, with potentially disastrous consequences.

- Those who take insulin need to be warned of the dangers of hypoglycaemia when consuming alcohol. People around them should be aware of their diabetes.

- It is prudent to maintain blood glucose levels a little higher if they plan to drink a potentially intoxicating volume of alcohol; carbohydrate snacks should be eaten as well in such situations.

Alcohol has a well recognised propensity to impair recovery from hypoglycaemia.

Patients particularly prone to hypoglycaemia

Those with diabetes at the extreme of age are at particularly high risk of hypoglycaemia.

- *Infants and young children.* These groups are vulnerable due to the irregularity of meals and unpredictable exercise. Those in this age group are prone to nocturnal episodes partly because over 12 h often separates their evening meal from breakfast. One study reported rates of hypoglycaemia of up to 70 per cent in an unselected group of children attending a hospital clinic, who remained asleep despite profound nocturnal hypoglycaemia. The developing brain may be especially vulnerable to the damaging effects of hypoglycaemia. There is evidence that severe and repeated hypoglycaemia in early childhood can result in developmental delay and measurable defects in cognitive function. Both parents and health care professionals responsible for the care of young children with diabetes face considerable difficulties in reconciling the desire for tight metabolic control with the threat of hypoglycaemia. Rapid acting insulin analogues have been used post-prandially with some success and there is a growing trend to multiple injections or insulin pumps, specifically to reduce the risk of hypoglycaemia.

- *Elderly patients.* The elderly exhibit diminished sensitivity to catecholamines as well as a less prominent sympatho-adrenal response. Symptoms of hypoglycaemia are often less specific and coupled with the tendency of others to attribute confusion and abnormal behaviour to cerebrovascular disease increases their vulnerability to hypoglycaemic episodes. Since near normoglycaemia has uncertain long-term benefit in this age group, it seems sensible to aim for less stringent levels of glycaemic control to prevent unnecessary hypoglycaemia.

> Patients at the extremes of age are more vulnerable to the
> adverse effects of hypoglycaemia.

Does the species of insulin affect the risk of hypoglycaemia?

The question of whether human insulin might contribute to hypoglycaemia unawareness was raised during the 1980s. The development of recombinant insulin of human structure resulted in its widespread introduction to many patients who previously been using animal insulin without problems. A minority complained vociferously of different problems including a major reduction in hypoglycaemic warning signs, which improved when they were transferred back to animal insulin. However, repeated studies have failed either to confirm a consistent reduction in physiological responses and symptoms in those on human insulin or identify any convincing mechanisms. Furthermore, the concerns were confined to only a few countries such as the UK and Switzerland. The introduction of human insulin in others such as the USA and Germany produced few problems. To some, the most likely explanation is that the time of transfer coincided with attempts to tighten glycaemic control, and it was this that led to a loss of hypoglycaemic warning. Others have suggested that an increased rate of asymptomatic nocturnal hypoglycaemia due to differences in insulin kinetics could have caused a reduction in autonomic symptoms. Many years later, the question remains unresolved and it now seems unlikely that a study with sufficient power will ever be mounted. It is ironic that recombinant technology has now resulted in the development of both short- and long-acting insulin analogues whose chief benefit is to reduce the incidence of hypoglycaemia.

> The controversial issue of insulin species and risk of hypoglycaemia remains unresolved.

Diagnosis and management

In a patient known to have insulin-treated diabetes with features suggestive of hypoglycaemia,

- rapidly measure capillary blood glucose at the bedside.

- Take venous blood (in a fluoride oxalate tube) for confirmation of the diagnosis by an accredited laboratory.

- In the uncommon situation wherein the patient is not known to have diabetes, take 10 mL plasma simultaneously and ask the laboratory to freeze at $-20°C$; this allows plasma insulin and/or sulphonylurea concentrations to be measured subsequently if an insulinoma needs to be excluded or sulphonylurea-induced hypoglycaemia (see Chapter 5) is suspected; certain tumours are associated with hypoglycaemia with appropriately suppressed insulin concentrations. Other potential causes of spontaneous hypoglycaemia include

  - excessive alcohol consumption, especially in children or in the absence of carbohydrate intake

  - severe liver disease

  - hypoadrenalism – primary or secondary e.g. hypopituitarism.

If the patient is able to maintain an airway give oral glucose ideally in liquid form, e.g. a proprietary glucose drink. Preparations in gelform, e.g. Hypostop®, may also be useful. If patients are unable to take anything orally then give either i.m. glucagon or i.v. dextrose.

Glucagon. This is the initial treatment of choice as it can be given by both paramedics and nursing staff. Give 0.5–1.0 mg i.m.; it can cause vomiting, particularly in children and at higher doses in adults. Give i.v. dextrose if there has been no response after 10 min. It is important to ensure that oral carbohydrate is taken after the patient regains consciousness to prevent early relapse.

Intravenous dextrose. Give as 20–30 mL of 50 per cent dextrose into a large forearm vein, which should be flushed afterwards with saline to reduce the chances of thrombophlebitis. Do not overtreat. Start an i.v. infusion of 10 per cent dextrose in those who fail to maintain their blood glucose at normal levels or who do not regain consciousness.

Other measures. Prolonged coma, i.e. >60 min, raises the possibility of cerebral damage. Maintain blood glucose at around 10 mmol/L. Dexamethasone is often given to reduce cerebral oedema, although there are no published data establishing benefit. Even prolonged coma lasting for many hours has been followed by an apparently full recovery. Those who make a rapid recovery and whose blood glucose remains stable over one hour can be discharged from hospital, ideally in the care of a relative or friend. Consider the precipitating cause. If one can be identified, take steps to avoid further episodes, e.g. by reducing insulin dose, if appropriate. Inform the clinician supervising the usual care of the patient.

What do patients need to know about hypoglycaemia?

The symptoms of hypoglycaemia should be explained to all patients starting insulin together with the appropriate action they should take in response to such symptoms. It is still part of the educational policy in some centres to induce a hypoglycaemic episode in hospital shortly after diagnosis. This is difficult to achieve reliably and the symptoms produced in this artificial situation are often different from those experienced at home. Since poorly supervised attempts have occasionally resulted in permanent brain damage and death such a policy seems of little value and should be abandoned.

Many patients fear the risks and results of hypoglycaemia more than microvascular complications and a discussion of these issues should be part of any structured education programme. Individuals and their families should be told that mild hypoglycaemia is an inevitable part of life for anyone maintaining tight glucose control and that even severe episodes rarely cause permanent harm. The families of those with insulin-treated diabetes also need to know how to treat a severe episode, including the use of glucagon.

The problem of hypoglycaemia in insulin-treated patients will only be solved by the still distant prospect of new methods of insulin delivery. However, the present situation may be alleviated by the imminent development of reliable continuous glucose sensors incorporating an alarm, e.g. to wake patients before they develop severe nocturnal hypoglycaemia. Until then, we need to ensure that patients are realistically informed about the risks and that they possess the skills to manage their insulin treatment effectively.

> Steps should be taken to avoid recurrence of severe insulin-induced hypoglycaemia wherever possible.

Further reading

Cranston I, Lomas J, Maran A, Macdonald IA and Amiel SA. Restoration of hypoglycaemia unawareness in patients with long-duration insulin-dependent diabetes. *Lancet* 1994; **344**: 283–287.

Cryer PE. Hierarchy of physiological responses to hypoglycemia: relevance to clinical hypoglycemia in type I (insulin dependent) diabetes mellitus. *Hormone Metab Res* 1997; **29**: 92–96.

Davis SN, Shavers C, Costa F and Mosqueda-Garcia R. Role of cortisol in the pathogenesis of deficient counterregulation after antecedent hypoglycemia in normal humans. *J Clin Invest* 1996; **98**: 680–691.

Diabetes Control and Complications Trial Research Group. The effect of intensive treatment of diabetes on the development and progression of long-term complications in insulin-dependent diabetes mellitus. *N Engl J Med* 1993; **329**: 683–689.

Heller SR. How should hypoglycaemia unawareness be managed? In: Gill G, Williams G, Pickup J, eds. Difficult Diabetes – Current Management Challenges. Oxford: Blackwell; 2001.

Heller SR, Macdonald IA, Herbert M and Tattersall RB. Influence of sympathetic nervous system on hypoglycaemic warning symptoms. *Lancet* 1987; **ii**: 359–363.

Jorgensen LN, Dejgaard A and Pramming SK. Human insulin and hypoglycaemia: a literature survey. *Diabet Med* 1994; **11**: 925–934.

Matyka KA, Wigg L, Pramming S, Stores G and Dunger DB. Cognitive function and mood after profound nocturnal hypoglycaemia in prepubertal children with conventional insulin treatment for diabetes. *Arch Dis Child* 1999; **81**: 138–142.

Meneilly GS, Cheung E and Tuokko H. Altered responses to hypoglycaemia of healthy elderly people. *J Clin Endocrinol Metab* 1994; **78**: 1341–1348.

Pramming S, Thorsteinsson B, Bendtson I and Binder C. Symptomatic hypoglycaemia in 411 type 1 diabetic patients. *Diabet Med* 1991; **8**: 217–222.

Rovet JF and Ehrlich RM. The effect of hypoglycemic seizures on cognitive function in children with diabetes: a 7-year prospective study. *J Pediatr* 1999; **134**: 503–506.

Tattersall RB and Gill GV. Unexplained deaths of type 1 diabetic patients. *Diabet Med* 1991; **8**: 49–58.

5

Hypoglycaemia Caused by Insulin Secretagogues

Kathleen M Colleran, Andrew J Krentz and **Mark R Burge**

Summary

The sulphonylureas were introduced into clinical practice in the 1950s, their availability representing an early milestone in the treatment of type 2 diabetes. Sulphonylureas remain a mainstay of treatment. There are a wide variety of sulphonylurea agents with differing pharmacokinetic properties that confer differences in risk of hypoglycaemia.

Sulphonylureas work primarily by stimulating islet β-cells to secrete insulin; the sulphonylureas are therefore insulin secretogogues. As a result sulphonylureas, like insulin, carry a risk of hypoglycaemia, this being the main unwanted effect of these agents. Due to the wide availability of the sulphonylureas, intentional overdose and accidental ingestion and are not uncommon, particularly among children.

Emergencies in Diabetes   Edited by Andrew J. Krentz
© 2004 John Wiley & Sons, Ltd   ISBN 0-471-49814-9

Sulphonylureas are a causative factor in up to two-thirds of all hypoglycaemic events. Actual or potential hypoglycaemia is often the limiting factor in attaining target glucose goals in subjects with type 2 diabetes. In fact, retrospective studies report an incidence of up to 20 per cent for hypoglycaemia associated with use of these agents.

Severe sulphonylurea induced hypoglycaemia is a medical emergency requiring hospital admission. The elderly are at highest risk, particularly if food intake is compromised or hepatic or renal disease is present; care must also be taken to avoid drug interactions. Treatment with intravenous dextrose may be needed for several days, particularly for agents with a long duration of action. The somatostatin analogue, octreotide, may be a useful adjunct to dextrose. Mortality related to sulphonylurea-induced hypoglycaemia is not insignificant, with case-fatality rates approaching 10 per cent.

Pathophysiology

All of the sulphonylureas are associated with a risk of hypogly-caemia. The mechanism of hypoglycaemia is related to the mechanism of action and the pharmacodynamic properties of the drugs. As shown in Figure 5.1, sulphonylureas work by increasing insulin availability through a multi-step process. They initially bind to the sulphonylurea receptor located on the plasma membrane of the islet β-cell. Upon binding to the receptor, an adenosine-phosphate-dependent potassium channel is inhibited. This in turn leads to depolarisation of the cell membrane. Subsequently, calcium channels open and changes in calcium flux result in the release of preformed insulin from the cell.

Sulphonylureas stimulate insulin secretion from islet β-cells; all sulphonylureas have the potential to cause hypoglycaemia.

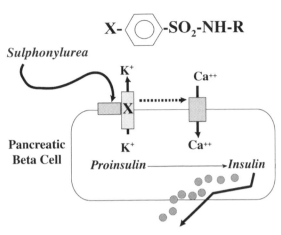

Figure 5.1 Schematic representation of the mechanism of action of the sulphonylurea agents

In patients with type 2 diabetes, sulphonylureas stimulate insulin release. The effects of the sulphonylureas are more pronounced in the setting of hyperglycaemia. In fact, sulphonylurea agents and glucose have a synergistic effect on insulin release; this can become a limiting factor in treatment. In the normal pancreas, insulin secretion is terminated once plasma glucose levels have normalised. In the presence of sulphonylureas, however, insulin release persists despite euglycaemia. Hypoglycaemia can thus develop if insulin release exceeds glucose availability. This occurrence can be observed in many settings, including excessive sulphonylurea dosage or lack of concomitant carbohydrate ingestion.

Another contributing factor to sulphonylurea induced hypoglycaemia is the presence of biologically active metabolites of the drugs. While the sulphonylureas are principally metabolised in the liver, many of the agents have active metabolites that are eliminated by the kidney (see Table 5.1). In patients receiving sulphonylurea therapy, the development of hepatic dysfunction or renal insufficiency can lead to reduced metabolism and delayed clearance of the drug. This is associated with prolonged exposure

Table 5.1 Pharmacokinetics of the sulphonylureas

Drug	Trade name	$T_{1/2}$ (hours)	Active metabolite	Renal excretion of metabolite (%)
Tolbutamide	Orinase Rastinon	6–10	+	100
Acetohexamide	Dymelor	12–18	++	100
Tolazamide	Tolinase	16–24	+	100
Chlorpropamide	Diabinase	24–72	+	100
Glibenclamide (glyburide)	Micronase Daonil Diabeta Glynase	16–24	+/−	50
Glipizide	Glucotrol Glibenese	12–16	−	85
Glipizide GITS	Glucotrol XL	12–16	−	85
Glimepiride	Amaryl	24	+	60
Gliclazide	Diamicron	10–20	−	60–70
Gliclazide MR	Diamicron MR	30–120	−	60–70

Trade names may differ between countries, as may the availabity of certain drugs or preparations.

of the islet β-cells to sulphonylurea, and the resultant hyperinsu-linaemia may be followed by hypoglycaemia. Sulphonylureas with longer half-lives and/or active metabolites are more likely to cause hypoglycaemia compared with agents that do not have these pro-perties. Drugs with these properties include chlorpropramide (no longer used in the UK) and the most popular sulphonylurea in the USA, glibenclamide (glyburide). The recently introduced once-daily sulphonylureas, glimepiride and gliclazide MR (not available in the USA), carry a relatively low risk, recent head-to-head data suggesting a lower risk with gliclazide MR. Tolbutamide, a low-potency first generation agent, has a short half-life with a cor-respondingly low risk of hypoglycaemia.

> The pharmacokinetics of sulphonylureas is an important determinant of the risk and severity of hypoglycaemia associated with their use.

Table 5.2 Risk factors for hypoglycaemia with sulphonylureas

Renal insufficiency
Hepatic insufficiency
Prolonged fasting, e.g. peri-operatively
Acute or chronic intercurrent illness
Long acting sulphonylureas
(chlorpropramide, glibenclamide)
Drugs that interfere with the metabolism of sulphonylureas and
prolong their bioactivity (see Table 5.3)
Short duration of use
Elderly patients
Polypharmacy
Alcohol consumption

Other factors include the following.

- *Advanced age.* This appears to be an additional risk factor for sulphonylurea induced hypoglycaemia. Retrospective studies suggest that elderly diabetic subjects do not metabolise or clear sulphonylureas as readily as do younger individuals. Drug may accumulate in this population, leading to sulphonylurea induced hyperinsulinaemia and hypoglycaemia. However, one prospective study in otherwise healthy elderly individuals with type 2 diabetes did not find such an association. It may be that additional or concomitantly occurring risk factors, such as acute illness, polypharmacy, medication error, or ethanol ingestion, coincide to increase the incidence of sulphonylurea induced hypoglycaemia in elderly subjects. Risk factors for sulphonylurea induced hypoglycaemia are listed in Table 5.2.

- *Drug interactions.* Several drugs can interfere with the metabolism of sulphonylureas. This may prolong their half-life and result in increased insulin secretion, thereby increasing the risk of hypoglycaemia. Table 5.3 lists these drugs.

> Patients with renal or hepatic disease are at increased risk of sulphonylurea induced hypoglycaemia.

Table 5.3 Drugs that delay metabolism of sulphonylureas

Warfarin
H_2 receptor blockers
Sulphonamides
Salicylates
Ciprofloxacin

Sulphonylurea induced hypoglycaemia is not only a problem in individuals with diabetes. It is also occurs in subjects who do not have diabetes, and these agents have been used in suicide attempts by both diabetic and non-diabetic individuals. This is in part due to the wide availability of, and access to, these potentially dangerous drugs. In fact, people without diabetes may be more sensitive to the hypoglycemic effects of sulphonylureas than are people with underlying insulin resistance and impaired β-cell function. Additionally, prescribing or dispensing errors have occasionally resulted in the inadvertent administration of sulphonylureas to subjects without diabetes, causing hypoglycaemia that often requires a thorough medical investigation to uncover (see Chapter 4). Sulphonylurea induced hypoglycaemia in children is not uncommon. In fact, approximately half of all cases of sulphonylurea ingestion reported to US poison control centres occur in the paediatric age group. This is mainly attributable to the large number of sulphonylurea prescriptions written each year and the wide availability of these agents. A single sulphonylurea tablet ingested by a child can lead to life threatening hypoglycaemia and requires substantial evaluation, observation and treatment as described below.

Sulphonylureas may be ingested accidentally, especially by children, or used in deliberate self-poisoning by adults.

Meglitinide analogues

The risk of hypoglycaemia associated with the recently introduced meglitinide analogue class of rapid-acting secretagogues appears to be lower than that observed with some sulphonylureas; this is particularly relevant among patients with erratic meal patterns. Repaglinide is a benzamido derivative that is taken with meals. It has a short duration of action and does not stimulate insulin release in the absence of glucose. If a meal is not taken, the corresponding dose of repaglinide should be omitted. Repaglinide appears to be safe in patients with mild to moderate renal impairment, although caution is required. Nateglinide is an amino acid derivative that, like repaglinide, is marketed as a prandial glucose regulator. The rapid and relatively short-lived insulin secretion that these drugs produce, in the presence of adequate β-cell reserve, reduces postprandial glucose excursions; however, the meglitinides also lower fasting plasma glucose concentrations, repaglinide being more effective than nateglinide in this respect. Clinical experience with these drugs is as yet limited. An interaction between repaglinide and gemfibrozil has been reported with enhancement and prolongation of repaglinide's hypoglycaemic effect; this is thought to be mediated through interference with the drug's metabolism by cytochrome P450 2C8. While the risk of hypoglycaemia with the meglitinides appears to be relatively low, care is required to ensure appropriate use in order to minimise this possibility, e.g. when carbohydrate intake is reduced due to anorexia or vomiting. Combining a meglitinide with a drug from a different class of anti-diabetic agents, e.g. metformin or α-glucosidase inhibitors, will increase the risk of hypoglycaemia.

Repaginide and nateglinide are rapid-acting secretagogues that may carry a relatively low risk of severe hypoglycaemia.

Diagnosis

Clinical hypoglycaemia is characterised by Whipple's triad (Table 5.4):

- symptoms of hypoglycaemia
- low blood glucose concentration
- resolution of symptoms with the administration of carbohydrates.

Typically, symptoms of hypoglycaemia begin when plasma glucose concentrations fall below 3.3 mmol/L in healthy non-diabetic individuals. Central nervous system impairment occurs at approximately 2.8 mmol/L. The symptom complex of hypoglycaemia can be divided into neurogenic (or autonomic) and neuroglycopenic symptoms (Table 5.5). The neurogenic symptoms develop in response to counter-regulatory hormones that are secreted in response to declining plasma glucose concentrations, namely epinephrine, cortisol and glucagon. Neuroglycopenic symptoms reflect an absolute central nervous system deficiency of glucose substrate. Neurogenic symptoms typically arise earlier and with relatively higher concentrations of glucose, while neuroglycopenic symptoms occur with lower levels of glucose (see Chapter 4).

Individuals with type 2 diabetes can have altered thresholds for development of symptoms of hypoglycaemia (see Chapter 4). Specifically, those individuals with chronically elevated blood glucose may experience hypoglycemic symptoms at normal or even elevated blood sugar levels compared with individuals with

Table 5.4 Whipple's triad criteria for the diagnosis of hypoglycaemia

1. Symptoms of hypoglycaemia.
2. Low plasma glucose at the time of symptoms – measured using reliable methodology.
3. Prompt resolution of symptoms with administration of carbohydrate.

Table 5.5 Symptoms of hypoglycaemia

Neurogenic (autonomic) symptoms	Neuroglycopenic symptoms
Sweating	Dizziness
Tremor	Confusion
Anxiety	Fatigue
Palpitations	Weakness
Hunger	Warmth
Tingling	Headache
	Difficulty speaking
	Difficulty concentrating
	Loss of consciousness
	Seizure

normal glucose tolerance. On the other hand, individuals with recurrent hypoglycaemia secondary to tight glucose control may not experience symptoms of hypoglycaemia until blood glucose is significantly decreased. This occurrence is probably a result of adaptation by the brain to ambient glucose levels (see Chapter 4). Thus, it might be more useful to think of hypoglycaemic symptoms in terms of glycaemic threshold rather than absolute glucose concentration. The glycaemic threshold differs between individuals and is lowered by the occurrence of recent hypoglycaemic episodes. As such, it is common for individuals with newly diagnosed diabetes to experience symptoms of hypoglycaemia shortly after they are started on pharmacotherapy for diabetes. In other words, because of the acute lowering of blood glucose that occurs with the institution of therapy, patients may develop symptoms without overt hypoglycaemia in this setting. Other patients with type 2 diabetes report hypoglycaemic symptoms despite normal blood glucose concentrations that improve with the ingestion of food. These symptoms are usually neurogenic in nature and represent examples of subjective hypoglycaemia that do not fully fulfil Whipple's triad.

Clinically significant hypoglycaemia is poorly defined. Based on the above information, we propose the following definition of

Table 5.6   Classification of causes of hypoglycaemia

Hyperinsulinaemic hypoglycaemia	Hypoinsulinaemic hypoglycaemia
Excessive insulin dose; mismatch to requirements	Insulin antibodies; rare with modern monocomponent and recombinant insulin preparations
Sulphonylureas	Reactive hypoglycaemia; uncommon
Insulinoma (may be inappropriate non-suppression of insulin secretion rather than overt hyperinsulinaemia; proinsulin excess	Short bowel syndrome
	Mesothelial tumours; primary hepatocellular carcinoma* Severe sepsis Adrenal insufficiency Wasting syndrome

*Due to insulin-like growth factor-2 production.

hypoglycaemia in patients with type 2 diabetes:

1. plasma glucose levels < 3.3 mmol/L in conjunction with the occurrence of neurogenic or neuroglycopenic symptoms of hypoglycaemia or

2. any plasma glucose concentration below 2.8 mmol/L regardless of symptoms.

Because the symptom complex of hypoglycaemia can be non-specific, confirmatory plasma glucose determination – using reliable methodology – is essential to verify that symptoms are truly attributable to hypoglycaemia and not to some other cause, e.g. anxiety. Once a diagnosis of hypoglycaemia is established, the aetiology of the hypoglycaemia should be ascertained. As shown in Table 5.6, the causes of hypoglycaemia can be divided into two main categories with differing aetiologies:

1. hyperinsulinaemic, e.g. sulphonylurea induced hypoglycaemia

2. hypoinsulinaemic, e.g. alcohol induced hypoglycaemia, Addisonian crisis.

Most of these can be ruled out by a thorough medical history and physical examination. It can sometimes be difficult, however, to differentiate among the hyperinsulinaemic causes of hypoglycaemia, and further laboratory testing is often required. In this situation, appropriate laboratory testing includes measurement of plasma concentrations of

- insulin
- C-peptide
- sulphonylurea.

These need to be obtained during the occurrence of symptoms of hypoglycaemia, wherever possible. C-peptide is a marker of endogenous insulin secretion. It is produced from the islet β-cells on an equimolar basis with insulin but is not cleared on first pass metabolism through the liver, c.f. insulin, more than 50 per cent of which does not reach the peripheral circulation. Plasma levels of C-peptide are increased by insulin secretagogues but are suppressed by the administration of exogenous insulin; clearance is reduced in renal impairment. Table 5.7 demonstrates the laboratory findings on the various causes of hyperinsulinaemic hypoglycaemia. Unfortunately, results of these tests are rarely immediately available and clinical judgment is frequently required in emergency management. Insulin auto-antibodies are common among

Table 5.7 Laboratory diagnosis of hyperinsulinaemic hypoglycaemia

	Insulin levels	C-peptide	Insulin antibodies	Sulphonylurea levels
Exogenous insulin	+++	−	+	−
Insulinoma	+++	+++	−	−
Sulphonylureas	+++	+++	−	+++

N.B. Plasma insulin and/or C-peptide concentrations must be interpreted in conjunction with the simultaneous plasma glucose concentration.

insulin treated patients; interpretation of their clinical relevance may be problematic. Because pharmacy error and accidental ingestion of sulphonylureas are not uncommon causes of hypoglycaemia, it is prudent that all medications that a patient is taking be checked for accuracy. Additionally, it is imperative to review all medications in the home in cases of hypoglycaemia in children, patients with limited cognitive capacity, or suicide attempts.

Management

The goals of treatment of all forms of sulphonylurea induced hypoglycaemia are

- prompt restoration of euglycaemia
- prevention of future episodes of hypoglycaemia.

There are several therapeutic modalities available to accomplish these goals, including

- elimination of drug from the gastrointestinal tract,
- administration of glucose – oral or parenteral – to re-establish euglycaemia
- administration of agents that will attenuate the release of insulin from the sensitized β-cells.

If a patient presents after a known intentional overdose of a large number of sulphonylurea tablets in a suicide attempt, activated charcoal should be administered. The role of activated charcoal in accidental ingestion of one to two tablets (such as usually occurs in children) is uncertain. In this setting, activated charcoal would be expected to be useful if the ingestion occurred within one hour of presentation. Induction of emesis is not recommended due to the risk of central nervous system depression associated with hypoglycaemia and the subsequent risk of aspiration of gastric contents. If hypoglycaemia is not initially present, serial monitoring of blood glucose is essential. Blood glucose levels should be checked every 1–2 h. Two factors must be considered in determining the duration of observation needed following accidental or intentional overdose:

1. onset of action of the drug

2. duration of effect.

Hypoglycaemia will typically occur within 8 h of ingestion in accidental or intentional overdoses. Thus, patients in these situations will require monitoring and observation for at least 8 h after ingestion. If no hypoglycaemia occurs during this time period, they may be released. Individuals with sulphonylurea induced hypoglycaemia due to hepatic or renal failure may require longer periods of observation, as the duration of drug effect may be prolonged.

If patients remain euglycaemic, they should be allowed free access to food and will not necessarily require intravenous administration of glucose. A desirable outcome can be anticipated as long as the blood glucose concentrations remain above 3.5 mmol/L. If hypoglycaemia develops at any time following sulphonylurea overdose, glucose administration is required.

• *Dextrose.* An intravenous infusion of dextrose (5 or 10 per cent solution) should be initiated and titrated to keep glucose concentrations greater that 3.5 mmol/L. Supplemental boluses of 25 or 50 per cent dextrose (20–30 mL, repeated as necessary) may be required intermittently (flush cannula to reduce risk of thrombophlebitis; Chapter 4). The patient should be admitted for overnight observation and glucose administration. Caution must be taken to avoid hyperglycemia with the administration of dextrose. As previously discussed, sulphonylureas have a synergistic effect with hyperglycaemia on the islet β-cell and may stimulate further insulin release and lead to persistent or rebound hypoglycaemia. The goal is to maintain plasma glucose concentrations between 3.5 and 4.5 mmol/L.

- *Glucagon.* If intravenous glucose is not readily available, 1 mg glucagon can be administered as a subcutaneous or intramuscular injection (see Chapter 4). Glucagon can also be used in the setting of hypoglycemic seizures. Glucagon usually results in symptomatic improvement within 10–20 min. The duration of benefit of glucagon is relatively short, lasting only 60–120 min. Because sulphonylurea induced hypoglycaemia can be prolonged in the setting of drugs with prolonged half-lives, decreased drug clearance (i.e. renal or hepatic impairment) or drug interactions, glucagon by itself is inadequate for the treatment of hypoglycaemia; dextrose administration is also required. Glucagon may be ineffective when hepatic glycogen stores are depleted, e.g. in the alcoholic patient. Some authorities caution against use of glucagon in sulphonylurea induced hypoglycaemia, since further insulin secretion may be stimulated.

- *Diazoxide.* This is a non-diuretic vasodilator, has been used in the treatment of sulphonylurea induced hypoglycaemia. This drug is an adenosine trisphosphate-sensitive potassium channel opener, which counteracts the effects of sulphonylureas on islet β-cells and will theoretically prevent insulin release. Onset of action is immediate after intravenous administration, and the effect lasts approximately 8 h. The drug must be administered in a separate intravenous line because it can precipitate in the presence of glucose. Unfortunately, side effects are common and include hypotension, tachycardia, nausea, vomiting and dizziness. Due to the side-effect profile, which is particularly undesirable in elderly patients with overt or subclinical cardiovascular disease and/or impaired autonomic reflexes, this agent is considered second line for the treatment of sulphonylurea overdose.

• *Octreotide*. This, as an adjunct to intravenous dextrose, is the drug of choice for the treatment of sulphonylurea induced hypoglycaemia. Octreotide is a somatostatin analogue that potently inhibits the secretion of several hormones including insulin, glucagon, growth hormone and gastrin. Octreotide binds to the somatostatin sub-type 2 receptor on the islet β-cells, inhibiting calcium channel opening, which decreases calcium flux; this results in greatly reduced insulin release, even in the presence of insulin secretogogues. Octreotide appears to be relatively safe in the acute setting. Side effects are mild, including nausea, headache, diarrhoea, fat malabsorption and discomfort at the injection site. Octreotide can be administered subcutaneously or intravenously. The onset of action is rapid, with a tissue distribution of 12 min; the half-life of octreotide is 1.5 h. Octreotide effectively ameliorates hypoglycaemia associated with sulphonylurea overdose and often decreases the need for exogenous dextrose infusion. These attributes may especially benefit patients with congestive heart failure in whom fluid volume overload is a concern. In the clinical setting, octreotide administration effectively reduces the occurrence of rebound hypoglycaemia following glucose infusion and may shorten hospital stays. Octreotide may be administered in doses of 50 µg subcutaneously or intravenously every 6–8 h as needed until hypoglycaemia resolves. An algorithm for the evaluation and treatment of sulphonylurea induced hypoglycaemia is presented in Figure 5.2.

All accidental ingestions of sulphonylureas in children require evaluation and observation in the emergency room. Studies suggest that if hypoglycaemia does not develop within 8 h of ingestion, then the risk of subsequent hypoglycaemia is low and the child may be released. If, however, hypoglycaemia occurs, the child should be admitted for continued observation and

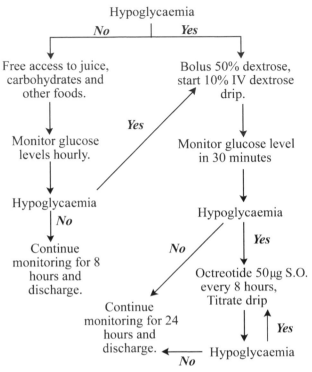

Figure 5.2   Clinical care algorithm for the evaluation and treatment of sulphonylurea-induced hypoglycaemia

treatment for at least 24 h to avoid relapse due to rebound hypoglycaemia.

Further reading

Burge MR, Schmitz-Fiorentino K, Fischette C, Qualls CR, and Schade DS. A prospective trial of risk factors for sulphonylurea-induced hypoglycaemia in type 2 diabetes mellitus. *JAMA* 1998; **279**: 137–143.

Burge MR, Sobhy TA, Qualls CR, and Schade DS. Effect of short term glucose control on glycemic thresholds for epinephrine and hypoglycemic symptoms. *J Clin Endocrinol Metab* 2001; **86**: 5471–5478.

Boyle, PJ, Justice, K, Krentz, AJ, Nagy RJ, and Schade DS. Octreotide reverses hyperinsulinemia and prevents hypoglycemia induced by sulphonylurea overdoses. *J Clin Endocrinol Metab* 1993; **76**: 752–756.

Herbel G and Boyle, PJ. Hypoglycaemia pathophysiology and treatment. *Endocrinol Metab Clin North Am* 2000; **29**: 725–743.

Jennings AM, Wilson RM, and Ward JD. Symptomatic hypoglycaemia in NIDDM patients treated with oral hypoglycaemic agents. *Diabetes Care* 1989; **12**: 203–208.

Seltzer HS. Drug induced hypoglycaemia: a review of 1418 cases. *Endocrinol Metab Clin North Am* 1989; **18**: 163–183.

Shorr RI, Ray WA, Daugherty JR, and Griffin MR. Incidence and risk factors of serious hypoglycaemia in older persons using insulin or sulphonylureas. *Arch Intern Med* 1997; **57**: 1681–1686.

Stahl M and Berger W. Higher incidence of severe hypoglycaemia leading to hospital admission in type 2 diabetic patients treated with long-acting versus short-acting sulphonylureas. *Diabet Med* 1999; **16**: 586–590.

6

Lactic Acidosis in Diabetes

Jean-Daniel Lalau

Summary

The classical view of lactic acid is that (1) it may be responsible for metabolic acidosis, mainly due to anoxia or ischaemia, to which diabetic subjects are particularly prone, and (2) such lactic acidosis is associated with poor prognosis. Indeed, blood lactate concentration is one of the best predictors of fatal outcome in critical illness. This observation contrasts with the fact that lactate is both a gluconeogenic substrate and easily oxidised, an apparent contradiction raising the question of whether excess lactate is deleterious, or possibly beneficial.

Current data are consistent with the notion that lactate production and related metabolic acidosis due to the stimulation of the anaerobic metabolism might be an adapted protective response. Diabetic subjects can also develop lactic acidosis due to accumulation of biguanides such as metformin. In clinical practice, this is typically referred to as 'metformin associated

Emergencies in Diabetes   Edited by Andrew J. Krentz
© 2004 John Wiley & Sons, Ltd   ISBN 0-471-49814-9

lactic acidosis'. This term is, however, confusing, because metformin use may be either the cause of lactic acidosis, for example, when renal failure leads to accumulation, but also, and more frequently, coincidental.

This raises two more questions. Regarding not only metabolic disorders, but also, and more importantly, clinical outcome, is metformin *per se* toxic? What role might metformin play in patients who develop lactic acidosis independently of, but coincidental to, administration of the drug? A recent insight is that no mortality is attributable to metformin alone, and that in the true metformin associated – as distinct from metformin induced – lactic acidosis, i.e., when both metformin and the associated disorder contribute to lactic acidosis, the metabolic and vascular effects of metformin may even confer some protection.

Lactic acidosis in clinical practice

Lactic acidosis is the most frequent cause of metabolic acidosis, with a prevalence of about one per cent among adult hospitalised patients. Lactic acidosis is of relevance to diabetic patients in two respects, one aspect being specific to diabetes, whereas the other is not. In the former category, causes of lactic acidosis include biguanide therapy, i.e. metformin accumulation. In the latter category, disorders of acid–base equilibrium are common in patients with critical illness, and critical illnesses are more common in diabetic patients than in non-diabetic subjects. Consequently, one should consider whether there is a difference between

1. lactic acidosis not related causally related to biguanide therapy

2. lactic acidosis induced by biguanides.

This distinction is relevant not only in terms of incidence but also, and more importantly, in terms of clinical outcome. Clarification of this question is relevant the management of overweight diabetic patients, in whom metformin has been recommended as first-line pharmacological therapy.

> Lactic acidosis is the most common cause of metabolic acidosis among hospitalised patients.

Following the classification of lactic acidosis by Cohen and Woods (1976) according to the presence or absence of adequate tissue oxygenation (Box 6.1), several excellent reviews have provided background knowledge on the diagnosis, clinical presentation, pathogenesis and management of lactic acidosis. We will therefore limit reconsideration of classical information, and focus on new directions.

Box 6.1 Distinctions among types and related causes of lactic acidosis

Classical distinction.

Lactic acidosis has been classically divided into either type A (anaerobic) or type B (aerobic).

- Type A is due to tissue hypoperfusion with reduced arterial oxygen content.

- Type B is due to a defect in energy metabolism indepen- dent of hypoxia. It includes common disorders (such as sepsis, hepatic failure, renal failure, and cancer), drugs or toxins (such as biguanides, ethanol, salicylates, metha- nol, ethylene glycol and niacin) and other conditions (such as strenuous muscular exercise, grand mal seizures and D-lactic acidosis).

Criticism of this classical distinction.

The above distinction is considered obsolete, given that restricted oxygen supply and metabolic factors often operate simultaneously.

Lactic acidosis independent of biguanides

Diagnosis

The definition of lactic acidosis is arbitrary (Table 6.1). In our opinion, reports in the literature and cluster analyses of laboratory findings in patients admitted to hospital for internal diseases support the use of this definition of lactic acidosis.

Table 6.1 Definition of lactic acidosis

- Arterial whole blood lactate concentration > 5 mmol/L
- Arterial pH ≤ 7.35

Note that lactic acidosis may co-exist with other causes of metabolic acidosis, e.g. diabetic ketoacidosis.

Pathogenesis

While hyperlactataemia refers to an increase in blood lactate, lactic acidosis indicates accumulation of both lactate and hydrogen (H^+) ions (protons). In fact, the formation of lactate from glucose neither consumes nor generates H^+. Although the metabolism of one molecule of glucose leads to the production of two protons, both go into the formation of lactate, such that:

$$glucose + 2\ ADP + 2\ P_i \rightarrow 2\ lactate + 2\ ATP$$

ADP = adenosine diphosphate
ATP = adenosine triphosphate
 P_i = inorganic phosphate.

It is actually the degradation of the ATP obtained that may cause excess formation of H^+ when tissue hypoxia hampers the recycling of ATP from its metabolites:

$$ATP \rightarrow ADP + P_i + H^+ + energy$$

Lactate production may also lead to metabolic acidosis in another manner, via the lactate/hydroxide (OH^-) exchange mechanism. The formation of OH^- from extracellular H_2O leads to entry of OH^- into the cell, where it prevents lowering of pH. Hydrogen ions are released in the extracellular space at the same time. However, pH does not fall if compensatory hyperventilation is sufficiently effective.

Theoretically, intracellular acidosis should exacerbate overproduction of lactate because the lactate/pyruvate ratio depends on the ratio of reduced to oxidized nicotinamide adenine dinucleotides:

$$[NADH][H^+]/[NAD]$$

This influence is, however, less marked than the strong negative effect of intracellular acidosis on phosphofructokinase activity, an action that acts as a protective mechanism during hypoxia by sparing glucose and, thereby, preventing the overproduction of protons originating from ATP hydrolysis. In addition, acidosis may improve tissue oxygen extraction, reflected in a shift of the oxyhaemoglobin curve to the right.

Prognosis

Lactic acidosis is still considered to have a high mortality rate. Indeed, blood lactate concentration is well recognised as one of the best predictors of a fatal issue in critically ill patients. Studies carried out in the 1970s showed a mortality rate of approximately 80 per cent for patients with lactate levels ≥ 5 mmol/L. This relationship has changed. In the 1990s, we observed the same mortality rate of 80 per cent for a fourfold higher lactate level. However, more important than estimating the isolated prognostic value of blood lactate concentration is determining what has caused lactate to increase in specific clinical situations. Because lactate may be metabolised and oxidised by most cells, the essential questions regarding the relationship between lactate and a patient's critical status are, in fact, whether

1. a high blood lactate level is the cause or the consequence of the severity of the metabolic disorder

2. the increase in lactate is a rescue mechanism that should be preserved.

Instead of being toxic, lactate may act as a preferred substrate for aerobic energy production during the initial stages of recovery from cerebral ischaemia or hypoxia (Box 6.2).

Box 6.2 Hypothesis for an adaptive role of the increase in blood lactate

- *A shuttle for energy metabolism between tissues*. When lactate is excreted by one tissue but oxidised in another, the latter tissue can be considered to carry out respiration for the former. When lactate is produced in excess, the higher the lactate turnover, the higher the energy metabolism of these producing tissues supported by the other tissues.

- *A role of sparing glucose metabolism*. The higher the tissue lactate level, the more glucose is spared for tissues with particular priorities (e.g. heart tissue).

- *A substrate for specific cellular function*. Lactate is an important determinant of cellular ATPase enzyme activities.

This idea is supported by the observation that lactate administration can prevent cerebral dysfunction during hypoglycaemia. The following mechanism has been proposed to explain these observations. During hypoxia, the ATP/ADP ratio is very low. When oxygen is restored to normal levels, lactate oxidation into pyruvate predominates over glucose oxidation, which necessitates preliminary phosphorylation to glucose-6-phosphate, an energy requiring process. In addition, for patients in critical condition, lactate can be viewed as a major metabolic substrate, *per se* or via its impact on glucose metabolism.

The view of lactate as an exclusively toxic molecule can be challenged.

Management

- *Vasodilators*. Drugs such as nitroprusside, which improve tissue perfusion, have been reported both to ameliorate and to precipitate lactic acidosis; their use has never been evaluated in a controlled clinical trial.

- *Vasoconstrictors*. The use of vasoconstrictive drugs, such as norepinephrine, is complicated by the potential of these agents to exacerbate ischaemia in tissues, such as skeletal muscle and liver, that are important in maintaining lactate homeostasis. Drugs that act principally by increasing cardiac contractility have not been rigorously evaluated in patients with lactic acidosis, but their utility may be mitigated by the negative inotropic action of acidemia *per se*. Despite decades of use, intravenous sodium bicarbonate has never been demonstrated to reduce morbidity or mortality in lactic acidosis and it may even be deleterious in some patients. Sodium bicarbonate is associated with several potential negative effects including

1. decline in intracellular and cerebrospinal fluid pH,

2. exacerbation of tissue hypoxia,

3. circulatory congestion,

4. hypernatraemia and,

5. hyperosmolarity.

Why this paradox? The explanation proposed – perhaps overly simplistic – is that CO_2 originating from sodium bicarbonate ($NaHCO_3$) diffuses more rapidly into the cells than its precursor.

- *Pyruvate dehydrogenase activation.* Finally, there has been much interest in the use of sodium dichloroacetate, which is an activator of pyruvate dehydrogenase. Consequently, dichloroacetate tends to eliminate lactate through the oxidative metabolic pathway. Nonetheless, although dichloroacetate has been shown to significantly decrease arterial lactate concentration and to significantly increase arterial pH in patients with severe lactic acidosis in a placebo controlled trial, this was not accompanied by improvement in haemodynamics or survival.

- *Other measures.* The efficacy of Carbicarb (an equimolar mixture of sodium bicarbonate and sodium carbonate) has not been confirmed in humans with lactic acidosis.

The above findings prompt us to concentrate on treating the precipitating cause of lactic acidosis and to optimize ventilation to compensate for metabolic acidosis. If lactate is a good metabolic substrate, hyperlactataemia should, in fact, be preserved (Box 6.3). Following this line of reasoning, the infusion of sodium lactate has been even suggested. Because lactate is both a strong and a metabolizing anion, sodium lactate provides a means of infusing sodium and decreasing the concentration of protons, which are removed along with lactate.

Box 6.3   Lactic acidosis: conclusions for new insights

The classical view.

Lactic acidosis is

- the cause of metabolic acidosis,
- primarily related to anoxia or ischaemia,
- and consequently associated with a poor prognosis.

From a biochemical point of view:

- rather than being toxic, lactate is considered a favourable metabolic substrate,
- lactate overproduction and acidosis may be a protective adapted response,
- management should, therefore, focus on treatment of the precipitating cause.

Lactic acidosis and biguanide therapy

Biguanides have enjoyed many years of use as oral anti-hyperglycaemic agents. Phenformin, however, was withdrawn in the late 1970s in most countries because of its association with a high incidence of lactic acidosis. Metformin has also been linked with this metabolic disorder, although less frequently (Box 6.4). This difference between the two biguanides warrants reflection. Is it simply limited to the incidence of associated lactic acidosis, or is the different frequency attributable to a fundamental difference in the nature of these agents?

Box 6.4   Incidence of lactic acidosis in metformin therapy

- The estimated rate is 1–9 cases per 100 000 person years, i.e. 10–20 times lower than that seen with phenformin.

- However, as metformin may either cause lactic acidosis or occur concomitantly with it, rates of lactic acidosis should be compared between users and non-users of metformin. This comparison was performed in a study of the US market before and after the introduction of metformin. This study found no distinguishable difference.

The above finding suggests a coincidental rather than causal relationship between metformin and lactic acidosis. However, given that metformin accumulation may lead to lactic acidosis, it would seem important to determine whether concurrent use of metformin, with or without accumulation, contributes to the course of coincidental lactic acidosis, especially with regard to outcome.

Relationship between metformin and lactic acidosis

The study of this relationship requires knowing whether or not metformin has accumulated. The best way of determining this is to measure the drug concentration in plasma, a measurement rarely performed in the literature (Box 6.5).

As a consequence of the high clearance of metformin under normal circumstances, and with the exception of intoxication with metformin, high plasma metformin concentrations imply both defective elimination and continuation of therapy. However, because the assay of metformin is not readily available, *a fortiori* in an emergency context, one may estimate the risk and extent of metformin accumulation based upon its pharmacokinetic characteristics (Table 6.2), the status and course of renal function, and

---

Box 6.5 An illustration of the importance of measuring plasma metformin concentration

This is the case of a patient with

- anuria (serum creatinine level of 350 μmol/L)
- lactic acidosis (lactate 16.3 mmol/L, pH 7.09)
- no interruption of metformin therapy.

A high plasma metformin concentration would have been expected, with the conclusion that the occurrence of lactic acidosis was secondary to drug accumulation. In fact, the plasma metformin concentration was within the therapeutic range. What else could explain the genesis of lactic acidosis? The occurrence of renal failure was recent and secondary to cardiogenic shock, which was the actual cause of lactic acidosis in this patient.

Table 6.2 Pharmacokinetic characteristics of metformin

- Plasma half-life: from 1.5 to 4.9 h
- Metabolism: not detectable – excreted unchanged
- Elimination: rapid renal elimination involving glomerular filtration and tubular secretion with a clearance of four to five times that of creatinine
- Approximately 90% of the ingested dose is eliminated in 12 h

dosage and time of last metformin administration. It is also possible to measure metformin concentration in red blood cells, where the elimination is far slower than that in plasma, thereby providing better retrospective information.

Although a low blood metformin concentration can rule out the drug as the cause of lactic acidosis in specific cases, the measurement of metformin concentration does not provide a reliable threshold of metformin accumulation and related disorders. This is because high plasma metformin concentrations are not necessarily complicated by lactic acidosis. This means that associated factors necessarily play a role, which may be evident in the case of patent disease processes, or less obvious, as in cases of a latent defect in energy metabolism. This ultimately calls for careful analysis of the history as well as the clinical and laboratory picture (Box 6.6).

Box 6.6 Questions to address when searching for a link between metformin and lactic acidosis

- Has metformin accumulated?
- Are relevant associated disease processes present?
- If present, is organ failure primary, or secondary to a shock syndrome (e.g. renal failure)?
- Are metformin accumulation and associated disorders underlying factors, precipitating factors, or both?

Metformin accumulation may be either

- a precipitating factor, as in metformin overdose or acute renal failure (when there has been no discontinuation of metformin therapy)
- an underlying factor, as in chronic renal failure.

Similarly, system failures may be either precipitating factors, as in sepsis or in haemorrhage, or underlying conditions, as in chronic organ failure. Taking such factors into consideration should help in estimating the prognosis.

Prognosis

Lactic acidosis associated with metformin therapy is typically associated with a mortality rate of around 50 per cent, similar to that reported with phenformin. However, since lactic acidosis in critically ill patients also carries a poor prognosis, it is important to clarify whether poor outcome is due to metformin alone, to the associated disorders, or both. To clarify this issue, the outcome of lactic acidosis in metformin treated patients in whom plasma metformin concentrations were available has been compared with the outcome in patients who did not receive metformin. The prognosis was better in patients treated with metformin, even though the observations were earlier and, on average, the patients were older, were selected on the ground of lactic acidosis and not only hyperlactaemia and, more importantly, had a median lactate level almost twice as high as the metformin untreated patients. In the metformin-treated patients, there was no relevant difference in median lactate level between those who survived and those who died. There was even unexpected survival in many who had severe lactic acidosis (with a lactate level up to 35.5 mmol/L) and circulatory shock. It was concluded that prognosis of lactic acidosis is independent of lactate level in metformin treated patients.

In the same manner as for lactate, if metformin were toxic, plasma metformin concentrations would have been higher in the patients with poor prognosis. It appeared, on the contrary, that the majority of patients with plasma metformin at the therapeutic level or even lower had the poorest prognosis while the majority of patients with high plasma metformin levels survived (Figure 6.1). If

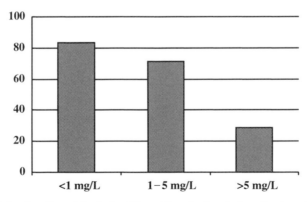

Figure 6.1 Lactic acidosis in 49 metformin treated patients with plasma metformin concentration available: mortality (%) according to plasma metformin concentrations (<1 mg/L, therapeutic or low; 1–5 mg/L, moderately increased; >5 mg/L, markedly increased) (Lalau, unpublished data)

Table 6.3 Differences between phenformin and metformin

Structural differences:

- phenformin has a long lipophilic side chain that mediates its binding to mitochondrial membranes, where it inhibits the major pathways of lactate disposal: gluconeogenesis and oxidation

- metformin has two small moieties that confer much less lipophilicity and, consequently, no marked inhibiting effect on oxidative phosphorylation.

Pharmacological and metabolic differences:

- phenformin is metabolised in the liver, and is associated with a well defined hyperlactataemic effect involving increased release from skeletal muscle and inhibition of oxidation

- metformin does not undergo metabolic transformation, or influence lactate turnover or oxidation. Its hyperlactataemic effect – actually minimal at the recommended dosage – originates from the splanchnic bed via lactate production by the small intestine after meals and/or defective lactate uptake by liver cells.

not lactate or metformin, what might account for a fatal outcome? The observation that most patients had at least one additional risk factor for lactic acidosis supports the hypothesis that concurrent diseases are likely to determine the outcome. Another point to consider is the difference between metformin, which has favourable metabolic and vascular effects, and phenformin. Although these two biguanides belong to the same family, they are structurally distinct, and the structural differences lead to differences in effects (Table 6.3).

The relatively good prognosis of metformin treated patients with high lactate levels may not be surprising. Indeed, as already stated, lactate may be metabolically advantageous. Bearing in mind that metformin treated patients with lactic acidosis may have very high lactate levels, the proportion of hyperlactataemia related to metformin with respect to that of an associated disease process may be relevant. Another reason may lie in various vascular properties of metformin (Table 6.4), many of which are unique,

Table 6.4 Vascular effects of metformin

• Macroangiopathy:	reduction in atherosclerosis reduction in thrombosis
• Microangiopathy:	improvement in haemorheology increase in nutritive blood flow reduction in vessel permeability
• Angiogenesis:	reduction in neovascularisation
• Haemostasis:	increase in fibrinolysis
• Oxidative stress:	reduction in oxidative stress
• Protein glycation:	reduction in protein glycation.

accounting for protection under ischaemic conditions. These vascular effects sharply contrast with those of phenformin, which has been shown to decrease cardiac output. While these differences provide a theoretical basis for the hypothesis that metformin may have beneficial effects in patients with lactic acidosis, this hypothesis has not been tested in a clinical trial.

Role of dialysis

Haemodialysis is classically considered to be the most efficient method, providing both symptomatic and aetiological treatment by eliminating lactate and metformin. This is actually a misconception. Lactate elimination cannot participate in recovery of acid–base balance since lactate *per se* is not an acid generating substance. Instead, the excess protons from hydrolysis of ATP during anaerobic glycolysis tend to be removed by endogenous buffers, which are regenerated through lactate metabolism. In addition, as already stated, lactate can be viewed as an energetic substance, and metformin is held to have beneficial metabolic and vascular effects. Thus, even if metformin can be readily dialysed, haemodialysis should only be considered for correction of blood volume and osmolarity in patients with anuria.

A critical analysis of the relationship between metformin and lactic acidosis

Because of the pitfalls listed in Box 6.7, considerations of the link between metformin and lactic acidosis in the literature are sometimes flawed. This was reflected in an analysis of 26 consecutive case-reports of so-called 'metformin associated lactic acidosis', in which lactic acidosis was in fact absent in four cases, not precipitated by metformin in another eight and of uncertain origin in two, leaving only 12 that were, in our judgment, precipitated by metformin.

Box 6.7 Summary of the pitfalls in determining the relationship between metformin and lactic acidosis.

- Overestimation of the prognostic significance of hyperlactataemia independent of metformin.

- Overestimation of the prognostic significance of metformin induced hyperlactataemia.

- Failure to measure metformin concentration in plasma.

- Failure to consider plasma metformin concentrations generating hyperlactataemia.

- Failure to consider prerequisites for the development of lactic acidosis.

- Failure to consider the prognostic significance of associated disorders.

- Failure to distinguish the effects of metformin from those of phenformin.

- Failure to account for different scenarios with distinct prognoses.

Conclusions

Use of the term 'metformin associated lactic acidosis', which commonly refers to all situations of lactic acidosis in patients receiving metformin therapy, is potentially confusing with regard to both pathophysiology and prognosis. Strictly speaking, this term should refer to metformin and concurrent disease processes as co-precipitating factors of lactic acidosis. Study of the link between metformin and lactic acidosis should instead lead to the distinction of different scenarios (Figure 6.2; Box 6.8). In true metformin associated lactic acidosis, for a given lactate level, the higher the

---

Box 6.8 Lactic acidosis during metformin therapy: new insights

The classical view of 'metformin associated lactic acidosis' is based on purely epidemiological data, which indicates an overall mean mortality rate of approximately 50 per cent.

It is more pertinent to replace this overall viewpoint by distinct clinical scenarios.

It is no longer acceptable to consider the association of lactic acidosis and metformin use in terms of mean mortality rates. Newly coined terms corresponding to entities of differing prognoses have greater clinical relevance:

- metformin unrelated lactic acidosis (without metformin accumulation): the prognosis is that of a serious, frequently life threatening underlying condition

- metformin induced lactic acidosis: the prognosis is excellent because metformin *per se* is not a toxic substance

- metformin associated lactic acidosis, with metformin accumulation and concurrent factors: the prognosis is intermediate, depending upon the severity of the under-lying and precipitating factors.

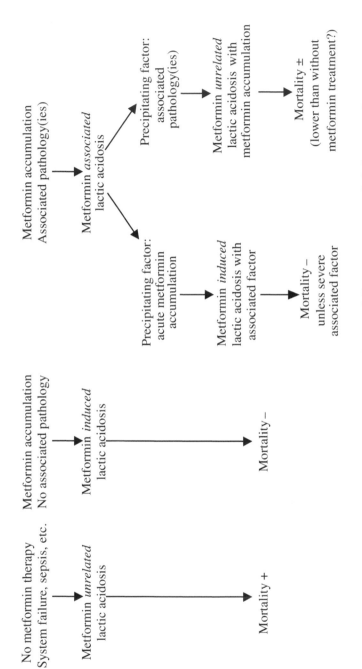

Figure 6.2 Lactic acidosis in metformin therapy: different scenarios and their prognosis

Table 6.5 Suggested revised contraindications and guidelines for withdrawing metformin

- Discontinue if plasma creatinine becomes elevated
- Withdraw during periods of tissue hypoxia, e.g. acute myocardial infarction, sepsis
- Withdraw for 3 days after i.v. contrast media is administered, and when normal renal function has been confirmed
- Withdraw 2 days before major surgery – use insulin if necessary – and reinstate only when renal function is normal and hypoxia, hypovolaemia, hypotension and sepsis have resolved.

Modified from Jones CG, Macklin JP and Alexander WD. Contraindications to the use of metformin. *Br Med J* 2003; **326**: 4–5.

degree of metformin accumulation, the lower the influence of the concurrent disease, possibly the higher the protective effect of metformin, and, ultimately, the better the prognosis.

It is clear from hospital and community based surveys that many patients receive metformin uneventfully even in the presence of traditional contraindications. Until such time that the contraindications to metformin are revised, the conditions listed in Table 6.5 provide a framework within which the drug should be used. The main contraindications were rigorously reaffirmed when metformin was introduced in the US in the mid-1990s. It remains possible that the low incidence of lactic acidosis among metformin-treated patients reflects, at least to some extent, observance of the main contraindications. There is scope for controlled clinical trials to clarify the contentious issues concerning the traditionally perceived safety record of this drug.

Further reading

Cohen R and Woods HF. The clinical presentations and classifications of lactic acidosis. In: *Clinical and Biochemical Aspects of Lactic Acidosis*, R Cohen and HF Woods, (Eds.) 1976, Blackwell: Boston. pp. 40–52.

Frayn KN. *Metabolic Regulation. A human perspective.* 2nd edition. 2003, Blackwell: Oxford. p. 339.

Fulop M and Hoberman H. Phenformin-associated metabolic acidosis. *Diabetes* 1976; **25**: 292–296.

Lalau J, Lacroix C, Compagnon P *et al.* Role of metformin accumulation in metformin-associated lactic acidosis. *Diabetes Care* 1995. **18**: 779–784.

Lalau J, Race J. Metformin and lactic acidosis in diabetic humans. *Diabetes Obes Metab* 2000. **2**: 131–137.

Lalau J, Race J. Lactic acidosis in metformin therapy: searching for a link with metformin in reports of 'metformin-associated lactic acidosis'. *Diabetes Obes Metab* 2001. **3**: 195–201.

Leverve X. Energy metabolism in critically ill patients: lactate is a major oxidizable substrate. *Curr Opin Clin Nutr Metab Care* 1999; **2**: 165–169.

Scheen A. Clinical pharmacokinetics of metformin. *Clin Pharmacol* 1996; **30**: 359–371.

Stacpoole P. Lactic acidosis. *Endocrinol Metabol Clin North Am* 1993. **22**: 221–245.

Vincent J. Lactate levels in critically ill patients. *Acta Anaesthesiol Scand* 1995. **39** (suppl. 107): 261–266.

Wiernsperger NF. Metformin: intrinsic vasculoprotective properties. *Diabetes Technol Ther* 2000. **2**(2): 259–272.

7

Management of Diabetes during Surgery, Myocardial Infarction and Labour

Aftab M Ahmad and **Jiten P Vora**

Summary

Surgery

Patients with diabetes are at increased risk of elective and emergency surgery, often as a consequence of complications such as advanced foot disease and the manifestations of atherosclerosis. Surgery stimulates the release of hormones and cytokines that antagonise insulin action and suppress insulin secretion. In patients with diabetes, this may result in hyperglycaemia and ketosis, depending on the degree of surgical trauma; even laparoscopic abdominal surgery can elicit a significant hormonal response. Metabolic decompensation increases morbidity in the diabetic patient via electrolyte losses, impaired wound healing and less effective cellular responses to

Emergencies in Diabetes   Edited by Andrew J. Krentz
© 2004 John Wiley & Sons, Ltd   ISBN 0-471-49814-9

sepsis. Inappropriate treatment with insulin or sulphonylureas may cause hypoglycaemia in diabetic patients fasted for surgery.

Intensive control of hyperglycaemia is necessary in high-risk patients in the post-operative period. Simple guidelines and good pre-operative planning are essential for successful management of surgery in diabetes. Patients with either type 1 diabetes, type 2 diabetes treated with insulin or patients with poor antecedent glycaemic control undergoing major surgery should receive a dextrose and insulin infusion; potassium should be added as required. This can be delivered as a combined infusion (glucose–insulin–potassium; GKI). More flexibility is derived by infusing insulin and dextrose (+potassium) via separate lines; the insulin infusion rate is adjusted according to frequent near-patient blood glucose monitoring.

For patients with diet or tablet treated type 2 diabetes, long-acting sulphonylureas such as glibenclamide should be changed to shorter-acting agents – or insulin if indicated – a few days prior to surgery; this will reduce the risk of hypoglycaemia, the clinical features of which are obscured by general anaesthesia. Patients with well controlled type 2 diabetes undergoing minor surgery should have capillary blood glucose concentrations monitored every 2 hours pre-operatively and during surgery; treatment is re-instituted with the first post-operative meal. Metformin should be avoided for all but minor surgical procedures because of the concerns about lactic acidosis.

Patients undergoing open-heart surgery with cardio-pulmonary bypass require higher doses of insulin, partly because of the use of high volumes of glucose containing fluids.

Myocardial infarction

Coronary artery disease is the most common cause of death in patients with type 2 diabetes and is an important cause in premature mortality in type 1 diabetes. Diabetic patients tend to have more severe and widespread atherosclerosis than age matched non-diabetic controls. Acute myocardial infarction has a higher immediate and delayed mortality than in non-diabetic individuals, cardiac failure and re-infarction being the main causes of death. The excess mortality among patients with diabetes has persisted with the introduction of effective treatment such as thrombolysis. However, diabetic patients derive benefits from such therapeutic interventions that are similar to or greater than those observed in non-diabetic patients; this reflects the higher absolute risk conferred by diabetes. Prevention of coronary heart disease, and other sequelae of atherosclerosis, is a high priority in patients with diabetes.

In a randomised clinical trial, the Diabetes Mellitus Insulin, Glucose Infusion in Acute Myocardial Infarction (DIGAMI) investigators used an insulin + dextrose infusion to achieve tight glycaemic control for the initial 24 hours on the coronary care unit in patients with an admission blood glucose >11.1 mmol/L; this was followed by multiple daily injections of subcutaneous insulin for at least 3 months. A control group received insulin according to clinical indications, a significant difference between the groups in the improvement in glycated haemoglobin levels becoming evident. Use of other treatment such as thrombolysis, aspirin and cardio-selective β-blockers was similar between the groups. Mortality was significantly reduced by 28 per cent ($p < 0.01$) in the intensive treatment group, with a reduction in absolute risk of 11 per cent at ~3.5 years; this translates into 11 patients treated with the intensive insulin regimen to save one life. Intriguingly, benefit was most apparent in a pre-defined subgroup of insulin-naïve patients, perceived as being at lower risk of mortality. Further evidence concerning the relative contributions of the early insulin–dextrose infusion versus subsequent insulin therapy is awaited from the DIGAMI 2 study. The latter trial may also determine whether twice-daily insulin is an effective alternative to multiple daily injections.

The cardiovascular safety of sulphonylureas, particularly agents that bind to sulphonylurea (SUR) receptors in cardiac and vascular tissues, has been an issue of controversy for decades. While no firm conclusion has been reached, some authorities recommend avoidance of drugs such as glibenclamide that can impair the phenomenon of ischaemic preconditioning (see below).

Labour

Diabetic women have a higher incidence of spontaneous premature delivery than non-diabetic women. Labour and delivery are potentially hazardous events for both mother and infant.

Insulin resistance increases during the second and third trimesters, necessitating an increase in insulin doses. All women with tablet treated type 2 diabetes should be treated with insulin during pregnancy. Blood glucose must be monitored carefully during labour. An intravenous infusion of soluble insulin should be commenced and insulin rate adjusted (usually 2–4 U/h) to maintain blood glucose levels of 6–8 mmol/L in all insulin treated women; to prevent hypoglycaemia, a 10 per cent dextrose solution should be co-infused at 125 mL/h.

Women with gestational diabetes who have well controlled diet treated diabetes do not usually require insulin treatment; nonetheless, blood glucose is closely monitored during labour.

After delivery, insulin and dextrose infusion rates should immediately be halved. The mother's pre-pregnancy insulin regimen should be restarted once she resumes eating.

Diabetes and surgery

The diabetic patient is at increased risk of requiring surgery for complications such as advanced foot disease and the manifestations of atherosclerosis. Often, such surgery is performed on emergency operating lists out of regular working hours when medical and nursing staffing levels are lower; in some countries, limited capacity may mean that surgery is frequently postponed, posing additional difficulties for patients who are nil-by-mouth. Even elective surgery is associated with hazards, being associated with higher rates of morbidity and mortality than in the non-diabetic patient. Major metabolic decompensation, myocardial infarction and infection are the main underlying causes for the high mortality during and after surgery. Diabetes is commonly encountered on general surgical wards; duration of hospital stay is often prolonged in patients with diabetes. Important contributory – but potentially modifiable – factors include

- sub-optimal peri-operative metabolic control

- imperfect monitoring of metabolic control during surgery and post-operatively

- presence of chronic complications, e.g. coronary artery disease or autonomic neuropathy, that render the patient with diabetes more vulnerable to adverse surgical outcomes.

Morbidity and mortality among patients with diabetes under-going surgery are higher than those among non-diabetic patients.

The use of uncomplicated management protocols, well planned pre-operative assessment and improved surgical methods has led to a reduction in mortality of diabetic patients undergoing surgery. Of note, recent data have demonstrated the benefits of intensive glycaemic control using i.v. insulin regimens in critically ill patients.

> Intensive insulin therapy can improve prognosis in critically ill patients with hyperglycaemia.

Factors adversely affecting metabolic control during surgery include

- diseases underlying the need for surgery, e.g. sepsis, atherosclerosis

- hormonal and metabolic responses to trauma

- nosocomial infection – more common in diabetic patients

- sub-optimal timing of meal delivery on wards

- starvation – may accelerate the development of ketosis

- certain drugs, e.g. anaesthetic drugs, corticosteroids etc.

Pathophysiology

As reviewed in Chapter 1, insulin is a powerful anti-catabolic hormone which promotes tissue glucose uptake, glycogen formation in liver and muscle, protein synthesis and lipogenesis. Catabolic hormones such as cortisol, catecholamines, growth hormone and glucagon oppose the actions of insulin by stimulating glycogen breakdown, gluconeogenesis, lipolysis and inhibition of protein synthesis. In non-diabetic subjects, surgical trauma results in increased catabolic hormone secretion, a relative decrease in insulin and increased insulin resistance in major target tissues such as muscle, liver and adipocytes; elevated levels of cytokines may exacerbate insulin resistance. The metabolic results of these changes can be intense catabolism, depending on the extent of surgical trauma, with increased glucose release and metabolic decompensation. Patients with type 1 diabetes requires higher insulin doses to counter catabolism. Those with glucose intolerance or type 2 diabetes are unable to increase endogenous insulin secretion sufficiently; insulin treatment may be required temporarily.

Management

Aims

The main management aims for diabetic patients undergoing surgery should be to prevent the following.

- *Metabolic decompensation.* This includes hyperglycaemia, keto-acidosis and hyperosmolar non-ketotic hyperglycaemia.

- *Hypoglycaemia.* Note that the diabetic patient under a general anaesthetic is unable to recognise or report warning symptoms of hypoglycaemia (see Chapters 4 and 5). Changes such as tachycardia that accompany the adrenergic response to hypo-glycaemia may be misinterpreted as being attributable to blood loss. Thus, careful and frequent monitoring of capillary blood glucose is the only means of detecting hypoglycaemia.

- *Delayed wound healing and sepsis.* Hyperglycaemia impairs cellular response to injury and infection.

Pre-operative management

One of the most important steps in achieving a good perioperative glycaemic control is a carefully planned preoperative assessment in diabetic patients undergoing surgery. This is best initiated well in advance of planned surgery, although in practice can be difficult to ensure.

- A careful general medical assessment should be performed, with particular attention paid to systems affected by diabetes. These include the cardiovascular system, renal function, autonomic system and blood pressure. Investigations should usually include

  o 12-lead electrocardiograph – even in the absence of symptoms of cardiac disease; exercise testing and coronary angiography may be indicated; note that clinically silent myocardial ischaemia is more common in the diabetic patient

  o chest X-ray, if any suspicion of cardio-pulmonary disease

  o biochemical assessment of renal function, i.e. plasma creatinine and electrolyte concentrations. Note that reliance on plasma creatinine concentrations may underestimate renal impairment, particularly in the elderly. Hyporeninaemic hypoaldosteronism associated with diabetic nephropathy predisposes to hyperkalaemia.

- It is important to liaise with the anaesthetist, who should be made aware of all diabetic patients for whom surgery is planned.

- Further assessment depends on whether these patients are undergoing minor or major surgery. The former includes day-case procedures such as upper gastrointestinal endoscopy.

Minor Surgery and Day-case Procedures

- Ideally patients should be admitted to the hospital the night before the operation, but if not possible than they should be dealt with as day cases and admitted early on the morning of the operation.

- Aim to ensure good pre-operative glycaemic control; since this may take some time to organise, the earliest opportunity should be taken to initiate changes in therapy. Liaise with the diabetes care team. Check haemoglobin A_{1c} and use the patient's blood glucose self-monitoring results to optimise anti-diabetic therapy. Targets of ≤ 7.5 per cent for glycated haemoglobin and pre-prandial capillary blood glucose concentrations ≤ 6 mmol/L should be sought, where feasible. In patients with co-morbidities, e.g. renal or cardiac failure, it may prove difficult to attain such targets safely because of the high risk of hypoglycaemia (see Chapter 4). This may necessitate adjustment of present doses of oral anti-diabetic agents and/or insulin; some patients will require the addition of insulin to oral therapy, or complete substitution of insulin for oral agents. While excellent glycaemic control is particularly important in the patient heading for major surgery (see below), minor procedures, e.g. angiography for aorto-femoral atherosclerosis, or digit amputation, sometimes require more invasive interventions because of complications.

Major Surgery

- All diabetic patients undergoing major surgery should ideally be admitted to hospital 2–3 days prior to surgery. If this is not possible then admit at least 24 hours beforehand.

- Replace long-acting blood glucose lowering agents such as glibenclamide with shorter-acting agents such as gliclazide or glipizide to reduce the risk of hypoglycaemia (see Chapter 5). Hypoglycaemia with agents such as chlorpropamide, no longer used in the UK, can sometimes occur.

- Avoid the use of metformin as this may predispose to lactic acidosis, particularly in patients with renal insufficiency, sepsis or hypotension (see Chapter 6).

- Monitor capillary blood glucose levels during the stay and optimise glycaemic control. Change from oral agents to insulin if control is inadequate (see above). For some patients already on insulin therapy, a change in regimen or insulin preparation may be required. For example, patients with inadequate control using twice-daily insulin may be usefully changed to multiple daily injections using short- or rapid-acting insulin before main meals, using a longer-acting preparation (isophane, insulin glargine, insulin detemir) at bedtime. In general, it is usually better to use smaller doses given more often in such circumstances.

- If possible, operate during the morning to avoid prolonged fasting. Although this is not essential, it is helpful to have the diabetes care team available for consultation in the post-operative period. Insulin withdrawal studies suggest that the development of ketosis (see Chapter 1) is accelerated in patients with type 1 diabetes who are fasted.

Operative management

Management of diabetes during surgery depends on factors such as

- estimating whether the patient can secrete adequate amounts of insulin
- duration and type of surgery
- whether post-operative ileus will be present.

Patients treated with insulin – whether considered to have type 1 or type 2 diabetes – should be assumed to have negligible insulin reserves; this is always the case in the former group and in the latter group is often the case for patients with diabetes of long duration. The implication is that these patients are at high risk of developing ketoacidosis if not treated with exogenous insulin in adequate doses. The clinical team, in collaboration with the patient where possible, must therefore assume responsibility for ensuring that sufficient insulin is provided to cover the hormonal response that accompanies major surgery. It should be noted that so-called minimally invasive surgery, e.g. laparoscopic cholecystectomy, is reportedly accompanied by a catabolic hormone response comparable to that observed with conventional surgery.

Minor Surgery and Day-case Procedures   It is generally agreed that a conservative approach is reasonable in these patients.

- Operate early in the morning, if possible.

- Omit breakfast.

- Omit the morning dose of oral anti-diabetic agents in patients with type 2 diabetes.

- Omit morning dose of insulin in type 1 and type 2 diabetic patients treated with insulin.

- Measure blood glucose every 1–2 h using reagent test strips in conjunction with a reflectance meter.

- Dextrose containing i.v. solutions should be avoided, unless hypoglycaemia develops.

This approach is widely practiced. There are no data from randomised studies to guide clinicians as to whether it is better to (1) omit medication or (2) to give the morning dose of sulphonylurea and to infuse 5 per cent or 10 per cent dextrose during the operation until meals resume again. Omission of medication has the advantage of an added degree of safety, since risk of hypoglycaemia is lower. For the majority of patients, the approach suggested will usually suffice.

Major Surgery

- Omit breakfast.

- Omit regular oral anti-diabetic drugs and breakfast insulin dose.

- At 0800–0900 h, an i.v. infusion of insulin + dextrose is initiated as follows.

  - Short-acting (soluble) insulin (50 U) is added to 50 mL saline (0.9 per cent) in a 50 mL syringe and delivered via a variable rate electromechanical pump (with built-in battery supply). Commence with 1–2 U/h, increasing or reducing the insulin infusion rate according to hourly blood glucose measurements; aim to maintain blood glucose concentration between ~6 and 11 mmol/L. An example of a variable rate i.v. insulin infusion regimen is presented in Chapter 1. Note that postoperative complications may greatly increase insulin requirements – 10 U/h or more may be required in the presence of severe sepsis. Thus, therapy must be individualised according to the clinical circumstances.

  - Dextrose (10 per cent) is co-administered via a Y-connector using a drip-counter at a rate of 100 mL/h, with appropriate potassium chloride (usually 20 mmol/L if the patient is normokalaemic with satisfactory renal function).

  - Advantages of this regimen include rapid and precise adjustment of the ratio of insulin to dextrose; disadvantages are risk of hypo- or hyperglycaemia if the insulin or dextrose infusion rate is incorrect or delivery is interrupted. It can be helpful to infuse insulin + dextrose for a few hours before surgery to permit stabilisation of blood glucose concentrations before the start of surgery.

- An alternative approach is to use a fixed ratio of insulin to dextrose. When potassium chloride is added, this approach is usually known as the glucose–potassium–insulin–GKI regimen.

  - 500 mL 10 per cent dextrose solution containing 10 mmol of potassium chloride (KCl) and 15 U of soluble insulin is infused at 100 mL/h.

  - Capillary blood glucose is measured every 1–2 hours reducing frequency if necessary, i.e. unable to achieve satisfactory control.

- Aim to maintain glucose levels between ~6 and 11 mmol/L.

  o If >11 mmol/L, change to an infusion containing 20 U soluble insulin, i.e. increase the insulin by 5 U in the new bag.

  o If <6 mmol/L, change to an infusion with 10 U of insulin, i.e. reduce insulin dose by 5 U.

- In elderly patients and patients with congestive cardiac failure, the standard regimen might produce fluid overload. In these patients a double strength infusion is prepared by adding 30 U soluble insulin and 20 mmol of potassium chloride to 20 per cent dextrose solution, infused at a rate of 50 mL/h.

- Caesarean section is usually an elective procedure and an infusion of dextrose + insulin in fixed proportions is reasonable (see below). However, insulin requirements can be expected to be higher in these patients due to pregnancy associated insulin resistance. Therefore, it is sensible to use 20 U of soluble insulin instead of the 15 U in the standard infusion. The pregnant diabetic woman already in labour who requires emergency caesarean section would already be on insulin + dextrose infusion; the latter should be continued during the procedure.

- A fixed dextrose + insulin infusion is also acceptable in emergency surgery. However, in cases where the last time of insulin injection is not known, care needs to be taken to account for the possible continued absorption of the preceding subcutaneous injection. In these circumstances, insulin + dextrose may be better delivered via separate infusion lines to permit rapid adjustments. Take care to correct any electrolyte disturbances.

- Patients undergoing open-heart surgery with cardio-pulmonary bypass require higher doses of insulin, partly because of the use of high volumes of glucose containing fluids.

Post-operative management

Minor Surgery/Day Case

- Patients should be re-started on oral hypoglycaemic agents with the first post-operative meal.

Major Surgery

- Continue i.v. insulin + dextrose until patient starts to eat when the patient's usual treatment can be re-started. Intensive insulin therapy in critically ill intensive care patients with blood glucose concentrations > 12 mmol/L reduced serious morbidity and mortality rate by 40 per cent in a recent clinical trial.

- Note that so-called 'sliding scales' of subcutaneous insulin are not recommended, since they use retrospective information to rigidly guide therapy. This is not to imply that pre-determined regimens should be unthinkingly enforced either. Rather, capillary glucose concentrations should be measured before meals and insulin prescribed according to food intake, knowledge of previous insulin requirements, likely insulin resistance etc. This requires experience and skill and is often a clinical challenge.

- Plasma urea and electrolytes should be measured 4–6 h post-operatively and then daily if the patients are receiving an insulin + dextrose infusion for more than 24 h; hyponatraemia is well recognised and can be largely averted by using 20 per cent dextrose in reduced volume (see above) or, where fluid overload is not a risk, by co-infusion of saline, e.g. 1 L every 24 h. Care should be taken to maintain normokalaemia.

To summarise, surgery in the diabetic patient needs careful planning and organisation to reduce complications and to improve mortality and morbidity rates. Using a variable dose i.v. insulin + dextrose infusion is a safe and widely accepted method to maintain satisfactory glycaemic control during surgical procedures. However, careful monitoring by trained staff and a rapid response if things do not go to plan are essential to ensure the patient's safety. The approach to managing diabetes during surgery is outlined in Figure 7.1.

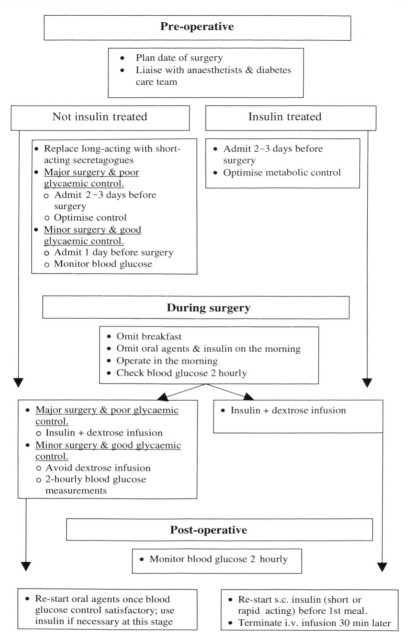

Figure 7.1 Protocol for management of diabetes in surgical patients

Diabetes and myocardial infarction

Diabetes is associated with a two- to fourfold increase in risk of cardiovascular disease relative to the general population. Cardiovascular mortality is doubled in diabetic men and the relative risk is even higher in women with diabetes. Data from Finland have suggested that mortality rates are comparable to those of non-diabetic people who have previously suffered a myocardial infarction. Acute myocardial infarction accounts for 30 per cent of all deaths in the whole diabetic population. More than 50 per cent of all patients admitted to coronary care units with acute myocardial infarction have some impairment of glucose tolerance. Epidemiological studies demonstrate an increased risk of early and late mortality in diabetic patients.

- Cardiac failure is the main cause of death following myocardial infarction in patients with diabetes.

- Re-infarction is also more common than in non-diabetic patients.

Accordingly, the prevention of atherosclerotic complications through aggressive management of modifiable risk factors including hypertension and dyslipidaemia is a major objective.

In patients with diabetes, myocardial ischaemia may present without pain – so-called 'silent ischaemia', which is thought to result, at least in part, from autonomic neuropathy. Atypical presentations of myocardial infarction include

- breathlessness due to worsening heart failure

- acute deterioration in glycaemic control

- vomiting or collapse

- acute confusion in the elderly.

A high index of suspicion is required to diagnose silent myocardial infarction. As mentioned above, subclinical ischaemia is more common among diabetic patients; this may be identified by a standard 12-lead electrocardiograph or by an exercise tolerance test.

Pathophysiology

It has long been recognised that patients with diabetes have severe and more widespread atherosclerosis than their non-diabetic counterparts. Traditional risk factors for atherosclerosis do not explain the high rate of coronary artery disease in diabetic patients. It is now widely thought that clustering of atherogenic risk factors is important. The metabolic syndrome of insulin resistance is commonly found in patients with glucose intolerance or type 2 diabetes. In 2001, the US National Cholesterol Education Program suggested clinical and biochemical criteria for the metabolic syndrome (Table 7.1). Other abnormalities, e.g. chronic inflammation

Table 7.1 National Cholesterol Education Program Adult Treatment Panel III criteria for diagnosis of the metabolic syndrome

- Fasting hyperglycaemia
  - glucose > 6.0 mmol/L
- Central obesity
  - men >102 cm
  - women >88 cm
- Hypertension
  - ≥130/85 mm Hg
- Dyslipidaemia
  - hypertriglyceridaemia >1.7 mmol/L
  - low high-density lipoprotein cholesterol
    - <1.0 mmol/L for men
    - <1.3 mmol/L for women

The presence of three or more constitutes the metabolic syndrome or impaired fibrinolysis (see below), are also associated with insulin resistance. Also of note, the 2001 NCEP report included diabetes as a 'coronary risk equivalent' in recognition of the high risk conferred by diabetes. The World Health Organisation has also produced a slightly different set of criteria for the metabolic syndrome that is not as readily employed in routine clinical practice. The metabolic syndrome is highly prevalent in the USA and many other industrial and developing countries, driven by adverse trends in body weight and lifestyle changes.

> The prevalence of the metabolic syndrome of cardiovascular risk factors is increasing in many parts of the world.

Atheromatous changes lead to impaired arterial relaxation due to reduced production of nitric oxide, a potent vasodilator; insulin resistance *per se* may be associated with endothelial dysfunction. Diabetes mellitus is also associated with hypercoagulability, the procoagulant changes on the endothelial surface favouring thrombosis. Platelet-rich thrombus in the coronary arteries is unstable and likely to rupture, causing acute coronary occlusion. Plaque in patients with diabetes may be particularly vulnerable to rupture due to a high inflammatory cell content and other adverse components.

The explanation for the continuing poor prognosis in the diabetic patient may lie, in part, in the secretion of counter-regulatory hormones that ensue after acute myocardial infarction; these result in adverse changes in cellular metabolism that are exacerbated by diabetes (see Chapter 1). Hyperglycaemia – secondary to acutely exacerbated insulin resistance and insulin deficiency – is accompanied by acceleration of adipocyte lipolysis, the latter resulting in release of non-esterified fatty acids (NEFAs). Myocardial glucose uptake and metabolism are reduced by insulin deficiency. Under these circumstances, the oxygen consumption of the ischaemic myocardium is increased by reliance on NEFA oxidation; this results in myocardial dysfunction that can be reduced if cellular glucose uptake and metabolism can be improved (see below). A chronic diabetic cardiomyopathy has also been described, which may contribute to the excess risk of heart failure after myocardial infarction in diabetic patients; the literature suggests that the size of infarcts is no greater among patients with diabetes.

Management

Once myocardial infarction is diagnosed in a patient with known diabetes, or indeed any patient with a blood glucose concentration > 11.0 mmol/L, the immediate steps in the management, in addition to analgesia and supplemental oxygen, are the following.

- *Aspirin.* This decreases the risk of reinfarction to a degree comparable to that of non-diabetic subjects. A dose of 300 mg should be chewed.

- *Thrombolysis.* This has been shown to decrease mortality in diabetic as well as non-diabetic patients and should be administered according to current criteria. However, the discrepancy in mortality persists in diabetic patients even with thrombolysis. Note that the presence of diabetic retino-pathy is not a contra-indication to thrombolysis, the risk of intra-ocular pressure being minimal and far outweighed by the benefits of reperfusion.

- *Percutaneous transluminal coronary angioplasty (PTCA).* Symptoms can be relieved immediately and at-risk myocardium can be preserved using this procedure; however, current practice in the UK is focused on revascularisation using thrombolysis as first-line therapy. The immediate outcomes of PTCA in diabetic patients are similar to those in non-diabetic patients, but re-occlusion has tended to be commoner in diabetic patients. A follow-up study of the BARI study (Bypass Angioplasty Revascularization Investigation) showed that diabetic patients who had previously undergone coronary artery bypass grafting

(CABG) had a better prognosis after subsequent acute myo-cardial infarction as compared with those who had received PTCA. Use of new anti-platelet agents and drug-eluting stents has reduced re-stenosis rates in diabetic patients. Specialist interventional cardiology services are a crucial component of high-quality care for high-risk patients.

Management of hyperglycaemia

It has become apparent that use of insulin to rigorously control hyperglycaemia after acute myocardial infarction is associated with major improvements in survival. The Diabetes Mellitus Insulin Glucose Infusion in Acute Myocardial Infarction (DIGAMI) study group treated patients with known diabetes, and those with a blood glucose values ≥ 11 mmol/L, intensively with an i.v. insulin + dextrose infusion for 24 h after admission and thereafter with multiple daily injections of insulin for a minimum period of 3 months. Patients in the intensively treated group received an infusion of 80 U soluble insulin mixed in 500 mL 5 per cent dextrose solution, initially at 30 mL/h for 24 h after admission and adjusted to achieve a target blood glucose range of 7–10 mmol/L (Figure 7.2). Careful monitoring by trained staff is required for safe implementation of the protocol, which carries risks of hypoglycae-mia. The intravenous infusion was followed by pre-meal soluble insulin injections given subcutaneously for a minimum of 3 months, wherever possible.

- In this randomised trial, the intensively treated patients were compared with patients treated with insulin only if this was considered indicated on clinical grounds. The 12 month mortality was reduced by 28 per cent in the intensively treated group; this improvement extended out to 3.4 years, the absolute reduction in mortality being 11 per cent (Figure 7.3). Interest-ingly, most of the benefit was observed in a subgroup of patients who had not previously been treated with insulin. For the total cohort, this translates into one life saved for 11 patients

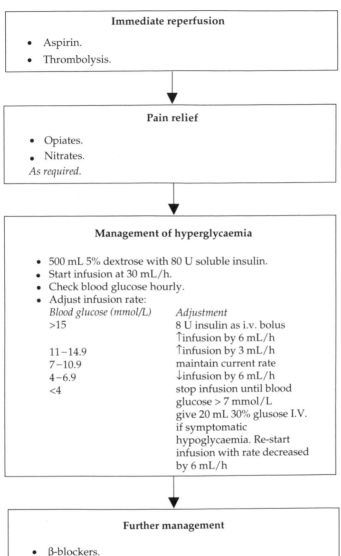

Immediate reperfusion

- Aspirin.
- Thrombolysis.

Pain relief

- Opiates.
- Nitrates.

As required.

Management of hyperglycaemia

- 500 mL 5% dextrose with 80 U soluble insulin.
- Start infusion at 30 mL/h.
- Check blood glucose hourly.
- Adjust infusion rate:

Blood glucose (mmol/L)	Adjustment
>15	8 U insulin as i.v. bolus ↑infusion by 6 mL/h
11–14.9	↑infusion by 3 mL/h
7–10.9	maintain current rate
4–6.9	↓infusion by 6 mL/h
<4	stop infusion until blood glucose > 7 mmol/L give 20 mL 30% glusose I.V. if symptomatic hypoglycaemia. Re-start infusion with rate decreased by 6 mL/h

Further management

- β-blockers.
- ACE inhibitiors.
- Statins – regardless of serum cholesterol concentration.
- Aggressive treatment of hypertension.
- Advise against smoking.
- Cardiac rehabilitation programme.

Figure 7.2 Management of myocardial infarction in patients with diabetes

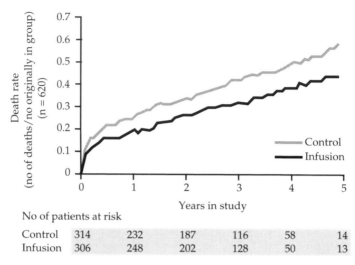

Figure 7.3 Actuarial mortality curves for patients receiving insulin–dextrose infusions followed by multiple daily insulin injections and controls. See the text for details. Reproduced with permission from Malmberg K *et al.* *Br Med J* 1997; **314**: 1512–1515

treated intensively; this compares very favourably with the effects of other measures, e.g. thrombolysis.

- Theoretically, some of the benefit of the intensive approach may have been due to a reduction in plasma NEFA concentrations, thereby reducing myocardial injury or improving myocardial uptake and metabolism of glucose. Another contributory factor may be the reduction in the sensitivity to circulating catecholamines and inhibition of the inappropriate neuroendocrine activation after infarction brought about by insulin infusion, thus lowering the risk of heart failure. A follow-up study, DIGAMI-2, aims to determine whether the benefits observed in the intensive treatment group were primarily a consequence of the early i.v. insulin + dextrose infusion or subsequent subcutaneous insulin therapy; it will also examine the efficacy of twice-daily insulin versus multiple insulin injections in this context.

> Intensive treatment with insulin reduces mortality in hyper-
> glycaemic patients following acute myocardial infarction.

- The cardiovascular safety of sulphonylureas, particularly agents
  that bind to sulphonylurea (SUR2) receptors in cardiac and
  vascular tissues, has been an issue of controversy for decades.
  While no firm conclusion has been reached, some authorities
  recommend avoidance of drugs such as glibenclamide that can
  impair the phenomenon of ischaemic preconditioning, i.e.
  reduced myocardial damage following episodes of prior
  ischaemic. Sulphonylureas release insulin by binding to SUR1
  receptors on the membrane of the islet β-cells, thereby closing
  potassium channels. Potentially disadvantageous interactions
  have been described between the anti-anginal agent nicorandil –
  which opens potassium channels in cardiac myocytes as a
  protective action – and glibenclamide; this is not observed with
  some other sulphonylureas, e.g. gliclazide. However, the
  clinical relevance of these observations remains uncertain. No
  adverse effect of sulphonylureas was observed in the United
  Kingdom Prospective Diabetes Study.

> The relationship between sulphonylureas and outcomes
> after myocardial infarction remain controversial.

Longer-term management

- All patients should be commenced on a cardio-selective
  β-blocker and an angiotensin converting enzyme (ACE)
  inhibitor, unless either is contraindicated; benefits of these
  agents are at least as great, and in the case of β-blockers even
  greater, than in non-diabetic patients. The small risks of
  reducing warning symptoms and recovery from hypoglycaemia
  (see Chapter 4) should not deter the use of cardio-selective β-
  blockers. Evidence is mounting that angiotensin II_1 receptor

antagonists are useful alternatives to ACE inhibitors for the minority of patients who develop a cough with the former class. Aspirin, 75 mg daily, should be continued, the optimal dose being uncertain.

• Serum lipids should be measured. Note that the very high risk of further coronary events in diabetic patients in effect means that *all* patients who survive a myocardial infarction should receive a statin, unless there are good reasons to omit this therapy. This view is supported by a considerable volume of evidence from controlled clinical trials and is endorsed by expert groups in the US and Europe. The primary focus on lowering low-density lipoprotein (LDL) cholesterol using statins is emphasised in the National Cholesterol Education Panel 2001. Doses of drugs that have been shown to be effective in clinical trials should be employed. The plasma lipid profile can be altered temporarily, with a risk that hypercholesterolaemia may be underestimated. Further assessment of a complete lipid profile, i.e. total, LDL and HDL cholesterol together with triglycerides after an overnight fast, should be performed at outpatient follow-up. More complex dyslipidaemias may require additional therapy; specialist advice may be needed. A mixed dyslipidaemia characterised the abnormalities in Table 7.1, is common among patients with type 2 diabetes. Other drugs, such as fibric acid derivatives, may be helpful, although evidence for the efficacy of this class lags behind the firm evidence base for the statins.

• Hypertension should be aggressively managed in diabetic patients; this often means therapy with drugs from two or three different classes. The target blood pressure is <130/80 mm Hg.

• Patients should be strongly advised against smoking; support should be offered, including pharmacological measures.

• All patients should, if possible, be enrolled in a cardiac rehabilitation programme; the benefit of supervised exercise programmes has probably been underestimated by many clinicians. Weight reduction, where indicated, and regular physical exercise as a long-term lifestyle modification, are strongly recommended, where feasible.

Secondary prevention measures after myocardial infarction include anti-platelet drugs, statins, tight blood pressure control, avoiding smoking and regular physical exercise.

Diabetes and labour

While this section focuses on management of diabetes during labour, some key points concerning diabetes and pregnancy deserve mention.

- Pregnancy should be planned wherever possible to ensure excellent glycaemic control at conception; this helps to reduce the rate of congenital malformations.

- Pregnancies in mothers with diabetes are associated with a high rate of late stillbirths; this remains incompletely unexplained. Late stillbirths are associated with maternal hyperglycaemia and fetal macrosomia. Macrosomia has implications for delivery, e.g. shoulder dystocia.

- Pregnancy is a state in which insulin resistance is temporarily exacerbated. This may precipitate glucose intolerance in susceptible women and has predictable implications for glycaemic control in women with pre-existing diabetes. Insulin resistance increases during the second and third trimesters due to hormonal changes associated with pregnancy.

- Women with type 2 diabetes or gestational diabetes that have sub-optimal glycaemic control should be treated with insulin during pregnancy. Women with well controlled gestational diabetes should measure their blood glucose six times per day on three days per week.

- Pre-eclampsia is at least two- to fourfold more common in diabetic than in non-diabetic pregnancies. Diabetic pre-eclampsia is associated with 60 per 1000 deaths compared to 3.3 per 1000 deaths in normotensive diabetic pregnancies. Vascular disease, pre-existing microalbuminuria, diabetic nephropathy, long duration of diabetes and poor glycaemic control are independent risk factors for pre-eclampsia. Pre-eclampsia is one of the causes of spontaneous pre-term labour and delivery, which has an increased peri-natal morbidity and mortality. Women with insulin treated diabetes (which includes both type 1 and type 2 diabetes) that antedates pregnancy have up to 25 per cent incidence of spontaneous premature labour and delivery. Spontaneous pre-term delivery is associated with antecedent poor glycaemic control and urogenital infection.

- The incidence of gestational diabetes, i.e. diabetes diagnosed during pregnancy, reflects factors such as age, obesity, ethnicity and methods of ascertainment.

Pregnancy is regarded as high risk in women with diabetes, posing hazards for both mother and fetus.

Pathophysiology

Maternal diabetes may affect the structure and function of the placenta. Fetal hypoxia, acidosis, placental dysfunction and hypokalaemia leading to cardiac dysrhythmias are the possible underlying causes for the higher incidence of late stillbirths. Excessive oxidative stress has been reported at delivery, which may also contribute. Impaired oxygen delivery to the foetus, due to a higher affinity of glycated haemoglobin for oxygen than non-glycosylated haemoglobin, may be another contributory factor. The contribution of intra-uterine malnutrition to chronic disease including diabetes and coronary artery disease in later life – the foetal origins hypothesis – is supported by epidemiological and experimental evidence. Tight glycaemic control is the aim in women with glucose intolerance during pregnancy.

Management

Fetal monitoring

- In view of the association between maternal hyperglycaemia and fetal hypoxia, foetal monitoring is important. However, the intensity of monitoring is still a subject of debate.

- In cases where labour is progressing normally, the woman has no diabetic complications and wishes to mobilise, intermittent foetal monitoring may be acceptable if the initial foetal trace has been satisfactory. Continuous cardiotocography (GTG) may not be essential but may be reassuring. Some obstetric units now employ telemetric CTG.

Time and mode of delivery

- Premature induction of labour for the fear of sudden death in late pregnancy is no longer practised.

- Delivery can safely be delayed until term or 39 weeks in diabetic women with good glycaemic control.

- The mode and time of delivery need to be individualised in diabetic women with pregnancy complications or coexisting severe diabetic angiopathy.

- In the case of planned labour the following may be necessary.

  ○ Intra-cervical application of prostaglandin jelly to dilate the cervix.

  ○ Oxytocin.

  ○ Amniotomy.

  ○ Fetal heart rate should be monitored continuously during vaginal delivery and pH measurements should be performed when indicated.

  ○ In cases of severe exacerbations of retinal changes and general obstetric indications, caesarean section should be performed.

Management of diabetes during labour

- Management of diabetes during labour and postpartum period should be planned and discussed with the patient; the outline protocol should be recorded in the case notes.

- Insulin treated women are at risk of developing hypoglycaemia during labour; capillary blood glucose should be carefully monitored.

- In cases where labour is induced, women should be continued on their usual diet and insulin regimen until labour becomes imminent.

- The full range of obstetric analgesia should be available.

- Once the woman is in labour, the following are required.

  ○ Short-acting insulin should be commenced and given through a syringe-driver infusion pump containing 1 U/mL of soluble insulin added in isotonic (0.9 per cent) saline (Figure 7.4).

Plan delivery

- Discuss time & mode of delivery.
- Discuss management of diabetes.
- Record outlined protocol in patients' notes.

Management of diabetes during labour

- Continue diet and regular insulin until labour imminent.
- Capillary blood glucose monitoring every hour.
- Prepare a syringe-driver pump containing 1 U/mL of soluble insulin in isotonic saline.
- Start 2–8 U/h of soluble insulin.
- Commence i.v. 10% dextrose infusion.
- Adjust insulin infusion rate to maintain blood glucose between 6–8 mmol/L.
- Less insulin may be needed during prolonged labour.

Postpartum management

- Halve the insulin pump and dextrose infusion rate.
- Discontinue both as soon as the mother starts eating.
- Re-start pre-pregnancy insulin regimen.
- Paediatrician should be present at delivery to monitor neonate blood glucose levels.

Figure 7.4 Management of diabetes during labour

○ 10 per cent dextrose solution should be constantly infused intravenously at a rate of 125 mL/h, which provides 50 kcal of energy per hour during labour to prevent hypoglycaemia.

○ Capillary blood glucose should be monitored hourly.

○ Insulin infusion rate should be adjusted to maintain blood glucose levels between 6 and 8 mmol/L.

○ Intravenous insulin requirements are typically 2–4 U/h in uncomplicated deliveries; insulin requirements may decline during prolonged labour. Note that use of β-adrenergic agonists (to retard pre-term labour) and parenteral dexamethasone (for fetal lung immaturity) can dramatically increase maternal insulin requirements; severe hyperglycaemia and even ketoacidosis may be precipitated.

• After delivery and in the immediate postpartum period, we have the following.

○ Insulin requirement normally decreases promptly to the pre-pregnancy levels after the third stage of labour.

○ Both the i.v. insulin infusion and i.v. dextrose infusion rates should be reduced to half of that required during labour.

○ Once the mother starts eating, insulin and dextrose infusions should be stopped; pre-pregnancy insulin dosage are recommenced with the first meal. Women treated successfully with oral anti-diabetic agents prior to pregnancy may be able to re-start their medication, if not breast feeding. Note that oral anti-diabetic agents are always replaced by insulin during pregnancy because of concerns of teratogenicity and inadequate metabolic control.

○ A paediatrician should be present at every delivery of a diabetic mother as neonates of diabetic mothers frequently have hyperinsulinaemia; up to 50 per cent develop hypoglycaemia and the neonates' capillary blood glucose should be monitored every 2–4 hours. Hypoglycaemia usually responds to frequent early feeds, i.v. therapy being largely avoidable.

For women with gestational diabetes, a follow-up oral glucose tolerance test is recommended at 6 weeks. Such women are at high risk of developing type 2 diabetes and 6–12 monthly follow-up thereafter is recommended. Contraception and planning of future pregnancies should be discussed.

Further reading

Diabetes and surgery

Alberti KGMM and Marshall SM. *Diabetes and Surgery*, in *The Diabetes Annual 4*, Alberti KGMM, Krall LP, Editors. 1988, Elsevier: Amsterdam. pp. 248–271.

Hoofwerf BJ. Postoperative management of the diabetic patient. *Med Clin North Am* 2001; **85**: 1213–1228.

Marks JB and Hirsch IB. Surgery and diabetes mellitus, in *Current Therapy of Diabetes Mellitus*, DeFronzo RA, Editor. 1998, Mosby: St Louis. pp. 247–254.

Mesotten D and Van den Berghe G. Clinical potential of insulin therapy in critically ill patients. *Drugs* 2003; **64**: 625–636.

Diabetes and myocardial infarction

Expert Panel on Detection, Evaluation, and Treatment of High Blood Cholesterol in Adults. Executive summary of the third report of the National Cholesterol Education Program (NCEP) Expert Panel on Detection, Evaluation, and Treatment of High Blood Cholesterol in Adults (Adult Treatment Panel III). *JAMA* 2001; **285**: 2486–2497.

Haffner SM, Lehto S, Ronnemaa T, Pyolora K and Laakso M. Mortality from coronary heart disease in subjects with type 2 diabetes and in non-diabetic subjects with and without prior myocardial infarction. *N Engl J Med* 1998; **339**: 229–234.

Malmberg K, Ryden L, Efendic S, Herlitz J, Nicol P, Waldenstrom A, Wedel H and Welin L. Randomized trial of insulin-glucose infusion followed by subcutaneous insulin treatment in diabetic patients with acute myocardial infarction (DIGAMI study): effects on mortality at 1 year. *J Am Coll Cardiol* 1995; **26**: 57–65.

Niakan E, Harati Y, Rolak LA, Comstock JP and Rokey R. Silent myocardial infarction and diabetic cardiovascular autonomic neuropathy. *Arch Int Med.* 1986; **146**: 2229–2230.

Riddle MC. Sulfonylureas differ in effects on ischemic preconditioning – is it time to retire glibenclamide? *J Clin Endocrinol Metab* 2003; **88**: 528–530.

Yudkin JS and Oswald GA. Determinants of hospital admissions and case fatality in diabetic patients with myocardial infarction. *Diabetes Care* 1988; **11**: 351–358.

Diabetes and labour

Buchanan TA, Metzger BE, Freinkel N and Bergman RN. Insulin sensitivity and B-cell responsiveness to glucose during late pregnancy in lean and moderately obese women with normal glucose tolerance or mild gestational diabetes. *Am J Obstet Gynecol* 1990; **162**: 1008–1014.

Girling J and Dornhorst A. *Pregnancy and Diabetes Mellitus*, in *Textbook of Diabetes* 3rd ed, Pickup JC, Williams G, Editors. 2003, Blackwell: Oxford. pp. 65.1–65.39.

Greene MF, Hare JW, Krache M, Phillippe M, Barss VA, Saltzman DH, Nadel A, Younger MD, Heffner L and Scherl JE. Prematurity among insulin-requiring diabetic gravid women. *Am J Obstet Gynecol* 1989; **161**: 106–111.

Hanson U, Persson B, Enochsson E, Lennerhagen P, Lindgren F, Lundstrom V, Lunell NO, Nilsson BA, Nilsson L and Stangenberg M. Self-monitoring of blood glucose by diabetic women during the third trimester of pregnancy. *Am J Obstet Gynecol* 1984; **150**: 817–821.

Index

Emergencies in Diabetes Edited by Andrew J. Krentz
© 2004 John Wiley & Sons, Ltd ISBN 0-471-49814-9

Index compiled by John Holmes

3